UNSPOKEN

UNVEILING TRUTHS OF OUR EROTIC NATURE

JENICE REVERS

AWARD WINNING AUTHOR

To your Sexual
Exploration
Enjoy xxx
J Revers

21-02-16

Published by JL REVERS LTD
Dalton House
60 Windsor Ave
London
SW19 2RR
www.jenicerevers.com

Non Fiction Self Help

Printed in the United Kingdom

ISBN: 978-0-9935156-0-6

Contents

Dedication

To all those who want to spice up their sex lives, harness the awesomeness of their sexual energy and enhance their relationship with their sexual selves. If this is you, then this book is designed to eliminate all anxieties and reservations you may have about asking for exactly what it is you want and desire in the bedroom and boost your confidence to unashamed heights.

Acknowledgements

The idea and inspiration for this book came about as a result of the energetic pulling of a community of people who want more from their sex lives and believe that life is supposed to be fun. Therefore, thank you to all of you who are ready to embrace and celebrate your sexual selves as well as those who are tolerant towards others' sexual expression. I would like to express my gratitude to editors, Joanna Oliver and Daniella Blechner for ensuring that this piece of work was brought to the highest standard for expectant readers.

Gratitude to those who continue to respect my freedom of expression and despite not being in full agreement with my stance, continue to support and love me.

Disclaimer - Please Read This

The content of this book is based on love and respect for both men and women, hence, not meant to communicate any feelings of a derogatory nature towards readers. It is quite erotic as it is aimed at engaging readers in a light-hearted conversation around their sexuality. There are no true stories depicted, none of the images contained in the book, relate to scenarios referred to, nor to any of its content or its practices.

This book is not intended to be a relationship manual; however, any increase in your sexual satisfaction will enhance the quality of your relationship. It is not a counselling or psychological tool and therefore does not address sexual trauma or any physical or psychological dysfunctions around sex and your sexuality. This is not a religious guide or moral code on human sexuality and there are no religious views held within this book.

Although anyone may find the practices, disciplines, games and understanding in this book useful, it is sold with the understanding that neither the author nor the publisher are engaged in presenting specific medical, psychological, emotional, sexual, or spiritual advice. Nor is anything in this book intended to be a diagnosis, prescription, recommendation or cure for any specific kind of medical, psychological, emotional, sexual or spiritual problem. Each person has unique needs and this book cannot take these individual differences into account. Each person should engage in a programme of treatment, prevention, cure or general health only in consultation with a licensed, qualified physician, therapist, or other competent professional. Any person suffering from venereal disease or any local illness should consult a medical doctor before practicing any sexual acts described in this book.

Prelude

AROUSAL

Honey, you may be slow but you're so sweet!
Take your time, honey!
Oh, I yearn for your irresistible sweetness!
I melt with indescribable pleasure as your
yumminess touches my lips!
Oh, oh, honey!

Oh, your warm moistness flow to my sacred places!
Lingering in my deep, dark crevices and curves,
Nurturing my vineyard of luscious, juicy fruits
Dripping, dripping, dripping,
Moist, moist, moist
Soft, soft, soft
Wet, wet, wet
Moist, soft, wet
Oh, oh honey!

As I feel the strength of your desire, your passion,
My breasts tingle, nipples swell,
Warm ache pulsating between my thighs,
In heated anticipation of your tender touch,
I erupt in ecstatic tremors
Awakened by your erotic love!
Oh, oh, oh honey!

– Composed by Jenice Revers

SEXUAL DESIRES IS FUNDAMENTAL TO OUR HUMANITY

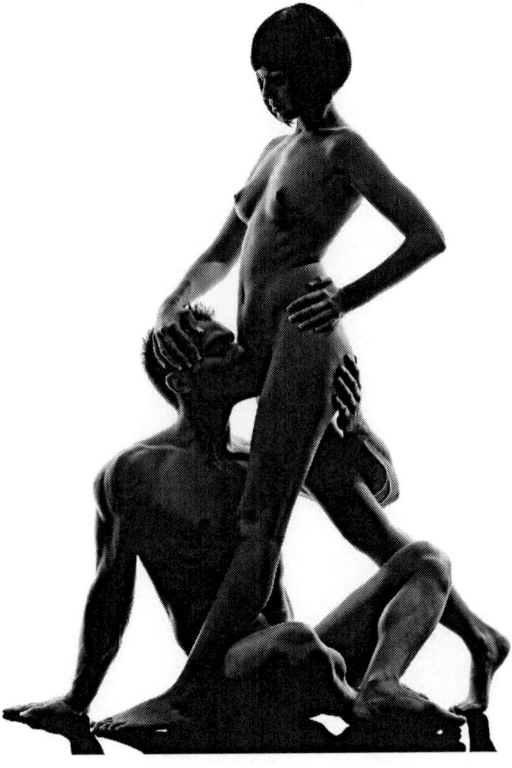

Introduction

How Could Something Feel so Good yet be so Wrong?

Sex is responsible for us all being here, so how come so many of us are afraid to talk about it or fully allow ourselves to enjoy it? Research supports the fact that sex has an abundance of physical, emotional, psychological and spiritual benefits. Not only can it cure that lingering headache but it's proven to be an awesome stress-reliever, self-esteem enhancer as well as wellness and wellbeing booster!

As a result of sexual intercourse, we benefit greatly from some life and health enriching, pleasure-generating chemicals, such as serotonin, oxytocin, dopamine and endorphins. Yet, it seems that we live in a society that appears to be doing everything in its power to regulate or repress sex and sexuality. Have you ever had a mean, angry boss who manages to continually get on their entire team of employee's nerves? Well, it is clear to everyone in the office when their boss is lacking any action in the bedroom. Hell yes! That's the awesomeness of sexual energy. This 'monster-like' boss would always transform into a smiley, amenable, approachable being after a couple of good nights' action in the sack.

In Tantric traditions, it is believed that our sexual energy—if harnessed—can be utilized to significantly boost our creativity, hence increase our productivity level. OMG! I guess workplaces need to consider giving both employers and employees f**k breaks throughout the day.

Who do you think enjoys Sex more?

I found the answer to this question on the internet when I was randomly browsing and entertaining myself with some sexual/sensual jokes.

"A man and a woman were having drinks at a business conference when they got into an argument about who enjoyed sex more.

The man said, "Men obviously enjoy sex more than women. Why do you think we're so obsessed with getting laid?"

"That doesn't prove anything," the woman countered. "Think about this: when your ear itches and you put your finger in it and wiggle it around, then pull it out, which feels better: your ear or your finger?"

~Author unknown

My hope is to engage you in an open, light-hearted exploration, in which we are free to talk about our sexual desires and the pleasures and ecstasy that derive from sex. I aim to enhance your sense of the sexual self, stimulate and awaken your sexual desires and empower your physical and mental sexuality. Over the course of reading this book, I will give you the opportunity to explore and identify your personal sexual fantasies or wish list, preferences, likes or dislikes. You will also identify your own journey of sexual disempowerment to begin to celebrate your sexual self with confidence and expression. Be aware that there are consequences to you being real about your sexual identity and feeling empowered. Should you progress to making this liberated stance, you are likely to lose some relationships or social status, for as we know, change is difficult for some people and especially when it relates to a change in another's identity – whatever it relates to. However, it is crucial that you consider the cost you would place on your personal/sexual freedom. Your sexuality is not just an insignificant part of you that you can forget about, yet continue to feel connected to self. With all that said: "Are you willing to continue this exploration of reconnecting with your awesome, juicy sexual self, and enjoy the heights of erotic pleasure and passion?"

Are you willing to continue this exploration of reconnecting with your awesome, juicy sexual self, and enjoy the heights of erotic pleasure and passion?

Yes_________ No_________ Not sure_________

If you are already feeling confident about initiating sex including when and how you want it, then take the opportunity to enhance your sexuality and experience erotic pleasure in the process.

This book is an awesome tool for singles and couples who want to spice up the action in the bedroom, on the kitchen sink, on table tops, on the toilet...or anywhere else this pleasure-sucking society will allow. It is also helpful as a catalyst to create a significant but empowering mindset shift if you associate sex with shame and guilt. You can start to appreciate this beautiful act as enjoyable, and therefore release all inhibitions and condemnations.

I believe that as people, our society—including religious institutions—have conditioned and socialised us to fear and be intolerant of differences. As a result, we appear to gain a sense of worth, righteousness and self-esteem in making other people wrong, especially about their sexuality. As I completed my research for this book, I was even more awakened to the double standards in our society. We have a society that celebrates contestants wearing swimwear in Beauty Pageants, whilst condemning images of Beyoncé and Rihanna as lewd and sleazy.

Are you going to allow a society who is guilty of such inconsistencies and double standards to determine how you embrace and express your sexuality?

I take a liberal stance around sex and sexuality as I believe that no institution has the right to regulate this personal, individual, intimate expression of life. I also believe that, as human beings, we are all on a journey to make sense of our existence and are seeking answers to questions about where we came from and where we are going. Hence, we find comfort and assurance in certain values and belief systems that we believe will secure a better quality of life now and in the afterlife. A major problem is that some sectors of society believe that their interpretations in regards to how we are to live are to be universally adhered to; if not, condemnation and an evil end await the unbelievers. BULLSHIT! There is no universal understanding of how we should express our sexuality. It is our choice to make.

I personally respect your sexual preferences, relationship types and status. Throughout, I will refer to sex between consenting adults. I would suggest that you be candid in your approach. If you want an 'open relationship,' don't pretend to be in a committed monogamous one. If you are homosexual, embrace your sexual identity and don't concern yourself with fear of rejection or isolation from family or society.

This book addresses societal beliefs or value systems that keep us somewhat repressed on issues of sex and sexuality. This is especially true for women, homosexuals, transgender and transvestites. I focus on building confidence around your body image so you can start to appreciate yourself as beautiful, sexy, sensual beings. Utilizing years of experience in counselling and psychology, as well as my own personal experience with energy sources, I will support you in your journey to discovering your own sexual story and empowerment. I will be cheering you on throughout as you discover, uncover and embrace your sexual identity.

Unspoken will help you to identify your 'sex' story and explore how it has influenced your sexual self. You will discover your ideal body image and explore your sexual attractions, as well as how they are manifested in your sense of sexual self. You will overcome the mental blocks surrounding your sexuality and explore your self-pleasure 'sex' story. My objective is to set a foundation whereby you are given the space and the time to fall in love with your physical sexuality and your sexual body parts, as well as to develop a relationship between your mental and physical sexualities. You will learn how to communicate with your sexual organs using sexually stimulating language to communicate. And all with confidence! Now is the time to identify and embrace your sexual fantasies. It's time to empower yourSELF!

I believe that for us to be sexually empowered is to be mindful of our own personal story, identity, and mental and physical sexuality. To be sexually empowered, we embrace our sexual selves and are confident enough to communicate our desires to receive complete satisfaction. Our sexual experiences are an essential part of our lives yet so often we overlook the importance of sexuality and our own sexual empowerment, in favour of what we think we should do.

Note that each person's sexual identity and desires are unique to them. Hence, a part of being empowered is to develop the ability to say 'No' if you are uncomfortable in participating in any sexual act initiated by another person. Sexual intercourse or play should be mutually desirable and pleasurable to all the people involved. Remember, sexual desires/fantasies fall at different points along the pendulum—from one from extreme to the next. There is a risk that your lover may or may not be into every fantasy and desire you may have. However, luckily, this is a world of variety and you are able to identify people who share the extreme nature of your desires.

You are sexy and sensual in different ways to others and sexual empowerment allows you to embrace your sexual self and share it with others with confidence.

As a woman who has triumphed over sexual trauma to realise sexual empowerment, I have struggled through past experiences that severely hampered my sexual comfort and acceptance. I have powered through the limiting conventional rules that stopped me from expressing my sexuality as an intimate part of my being and have found how to love and enjoy my sexual body and mind as an essential part of the whole. My personal journey has empowered me, and with my experience of counselling and psychology, I want to awaken your sexual energy.

How to work through this book

Throughout this book, each of the fourteen chapters begins with a short introduction to the topic. After reading through the material, there are a number of questions which are designed to get you thinking and explore your own experiences and instincts in a journal-like way. When facing each of these simple questions, write freely and write whatever comes to mind. Please note that throughout this book, I will refer to the person you are sharing your beautiful, sacred body with, as your lover. Whether you are in a short-term, long-term relationship or even dating, your lover could be your husband, wife, boyfriend, girlfriend, your date for the night or a regular date. I choose the term lover, as I am going to assume that whoever you are sharing your sweet, luscious body with, is someone who you are attracted to or have an emotional bond with. You might have one lover or many lovers and that's OK. It's your decision only—not your friends', family or the whole of society. Just ensure that you are open and honest about your position and treat each lover with affection and respect! *Agree?*

I will refer to tantric traditions or practices throughout; however, I am not an expert in this field, so I report purely from the position of what I have experienced firsthand or being an observer to demonstration upon others.

If you are happy with that, let's start our sweet, juicy love-making journey to Treasure Island! It is important to note that whilst we will be having a lot of fun, do consider your SEXUAL HEALTH- being responsible is just as important as a mind-blowingly pleasurable experience.

Before we jump headlong into sexual enlightenment, I have made a list below of some names used for vagina and penis; however, I will refer to the vagina as 'pussy' and the penis as 'cock' throughout. No disrespect meant or directed towards your sacred, beautiful, pleasurable treasure but from experience I realize that we are far more "naughty and kinky" in our minds than we would want to acknowledge to ourselves or be able to own up to with our lovers or others. So, I hope that with the use of these erotic terms, I will stimulate some sexual excitement and cause your sweet, juicy pussy or cock to pulsate somewhat whilst reading, resulting in a more pleasurable sex life. You are welcome to add your special names to the empty boxes and be sure to use them to spice up your sex life!

NAMES FOR VAGINA AND PENIS (Add to the empty boxes)

VAGINA				
downstairs		Pussy		Pink Fortress
	Cave of Wonder		Treasure	
PENIS				
Dr Feelgood	Dick	Buddy	Zipper Dipper	Sex Pistol
Love Shaft		Cock	Thrill Drill	Moby Dick

Chapter 1

Your Sex Story

BEAUTIFUL Me!

Sexy is Beautiful, Beautiful is Me
She is Desirable, Delectable, Luscious
He is sweet, sincere, succulent
Sexy is Difference, Sameness, Uniqueness
Sexy is together but sometimes alone
Sexy is being Beautiful and Me...

– Composed by Jenice Revers

What was your first sexual experience?

It is interesting to know the connection between your mental and physical sexualities. Your first sexual encounter will have a great impact on your perception about sex. Physical experiences, circumstances and encounters with people create memories in our mind hence creating associations and links. If our first sexual encounter was loving and affectionate and one of pleasure, then we will associate sex with love, affection and feeling good, however, if our first sexual encounter was one that caused us pain and suffering we may associate it with pain and powerlessness, shame and guilt. Our minds create associations and store thoughts, feelings and memories. It is important to know that thoughts can be rerouted and memories rewired with the help of a professional. Although your first experience of sexual feelings is a manifestation of both your sexual story and your body, your first sexual experience does not have to be the end of your story. Your initial sexual experience—how you expressed your early sexual feelings physically—has merely shaped your sexual story. This book empowers you now to create whatever story you wish.

Our pussies and cocks represent the physical manifestation of our sexual selves. It is important to note how your initial experiences represented your sexual self—both natural and learned—and how these experiences have further shaped your sexual story. Can you remember the first time you recognised yourself as having sexual feelings? What was your first sexual experience? How has it shaped your current sexual identity?

Many of us were raised in households where sexual expressions between our parents were non-existent or subjected to the privacy of their bedrooms, hence not seen or talked about. Some groups around us, institutional, family, friendship gave a negative representation of sex and sexuality. The act of sexual gratification is usually seen and talked about as 'dirty'. Sex became a "taboo" subject, which was never seen nor talked about. This lack of openness and lack of education, coupled with the shame associated with sex, I believe, has contributed to multiple wounds, such as unwanted pregnancies and other issues, such as the silence and shame surrounding child molestation and rape. We have also learned to fear sex due to the taboo category it falls into. It was the unknown. Girls were taught to be "good girls" and express no sexual desire at all. In turn, women have learnt to receive only and never to initiate their own sexual pleasure. As a guy, perhaps you were taught to be the dominant player in any sexual initiation. Sometimes this role as the dominator would include being aggressive and violent towards girls and women during sexual intercourse. Indeed our 'teachers' have taught us wrong and the time has come to take back our power because sex was meant to be a pleasurable experience with whomever you share your sacred, beautiful body with.

You may have been raised in a household where your mother and father had specific roles determined by their gender. You were probably taught that sex should only occur between a man and a woman. Your mother dressed in a particular fashion to represent her femininity and your father, his masculinity. However, perhaps you realised from an early age that you didn't fit into what was considered normal sexual identity—you were a boy who was attracted to other boys or a girl who found other girls sexy. You might have been a heterosexual boy who wanted to dress like a girl, or a heterosexual girl who wanted to dress like a boy... You might have been born with all the sexual organs and physical features of a girl but everything within said that you were a boy or vice versa.

Whilst some families and sectors of society might have been kind and accepting to your sexuality, I'm very much aware of how harsh some families and society can be. This comes from a fear of breaking the norm and being exposed to something different. Perhaps it is evident to you that you do not fit in with the norm in respect to your sexuality and, hell no, you were not meant to! You are a unique individual with personal likes, dislikes and preferences. Your sexuality is a choice! Take your power back and exercise that choice.

Be aware that you will need to be strong as you might be isolated by some family members, friends or some sectors of society. However, what you have lost in one area, the Universe will ensure you gain it elsewhere. Just be mindful and present in the moment, as a new soul-family and friends await. I have taken a similar path with my 'Faith', in that I have left a previously followed religious group to explore my own spirituality. In writing this book, I am aware that by embracing you and other people who are different to my previous religious beliefs, I am opening myself up to backlash and further isolation. However, that's cool with me, as there is freedom and peace in speaking and living in my 'truth'.

As people, we have come a long way through the hurts and pain to embrace and celebrate the awesomeness of our sexual selves. It is evident that we all have sexual desires and what better way to harness our energy than to explore and enjoy this sensual, physical and emotional act. It's time to embrace our awesome sexual selves!

Scenario

Shauntel is an active young woman aged 29. She was raised in a Christian household and her family are active church members. Shauntel knows that her parents have sex however, there was no evidence of their erotic desire for each other displayed or talked about within their home. Shauntel no longer attends church and feels restricted in regards to how she sees and expresses herself as a sexual being. She is in a relationship, yet she always waits for her partner to approach her for sex and, even when she is horny, she fails to ask for what she wants. Shauntel sometimes feels miserable with herself and her partner, as she struggles with the mental torture of not having her sexual needs met. She often has kinky thoughts of her boyfriend f**king her until she screams but instead, all she is getting is the 'good girl' missionary position. Shauntel's boyfriend, Cliff, respects her very much and sees her as a 'good girl', so would not dare mention to her his secret fantasy of having her talking dirty to him whilst having sex. Boredom sets in and their relationship almost resembles platonic friendship and they are both lacking the confidence to talk about their sex life...

Can you relate?

Yes______ No______ Somewhat______

Scenario

Karl is a 43-year-old medical doctor who is married to Lisa. He loves Lisa very much and they enjoy an active sex life. However, Karl has a strong desire to dress up in some of Lisa's clothing in the bedroom. He holds lots of fond memories of when he was growing up and how he would dress up in his mother's red lipstick and strut around the home in her high-heeled shoes. Karl doesn't feel like a woman; he just gets an intense sexual arousal when he thinks of dressing up in Lisa's clothing. He wants to talk to Lisa about this fantasy however, he doesn't know where to start. He doesn't want her to think that he is gay because that's not the case...not that he thinks there is anything wrong with being gay...

Can you relate?

Yes______ No______ Somewhat______

Scenario

Vanessa is a 33-year-old solicitor who works for a successful legal firm. She is single, however, she has previously dated other women. Her concern is that she has never felt like a girl or a woman. She has all the organs and physical features (breasts, vagina, womb etc.) but she feels like a man trapped in a female body. She is considering having reassignment surgery to change her physical appearance and/or hormone replacement. She assumes that her parents won't accept this. They know that she has dated other women and are OK with her being a lesbian but they won't agree to their daughter becoming a man. Nevertheless, she believes that she is an adult and it is her decision to make. She is aware that she might be isolated from some family members but she has a strong network of open-minded, liberal friends....

Can you relate?

Yes______ No______ Somewhat______

Reflection

What is your sexual story—your family and personal perception of sex and sexuality, and where does it originate? Is sex dirty, shameful, pleasurable, or beautiful? Are you allowing yourself to want it and to express that longing, or are you putting up certain barriers and stifling your sexual desires?

Chapter 2

Sexual Desires

"Women say us men only think with our penis...
ladies, don't be afraid to blow our minds."

– Author unknown

Do you desire sex?

Sex is natural, fulfilling, satisfying, beautiful, and pleasurable and so much more! But do you want it? And, perhaps more importantly, how do you want it? With family history, personal history, societal conventions and other causes, too often we deny ourselves and our sexual identities. We don't permit ourselves to want sex, and we become incapable of embracing our sexual arousal.

Arousal is our desire for sex and an expression of our sexual selves. Though we often think of it in a physical way, it is a very mental and personal thing and does not physically manifest itself further than our own behaviour and attitudes toward sexual experiences. This is especially so for us women, who sometimes struggle to feel our sexual desire because we are living stressful lives and are physically and emotionally exhausted. However, there are some self-nurturing things (i.e. time for resting and relaxation) that we can do to rekindle our passion. (We will discuss self-nurturing in greater depth later.)

I have been seriously playing around with some tantric and other practices of awakening your sexual energy to experience heightened pleasure during love-making. Therefore, I am aware there is a lot we can do to enhance our sex lives. If you have any concerns around feeling sexually aroused and you are clear that this is not medical or in relation to do with the impact of trauma around sex, I suggest that you work on your thoughts and physical stimulation to get your sweet sexual juices flowing. If you are dating or in a long-term relationship, you could explore reading erotica or watch hot love-making scenes in films or porn with your lover to fire up the sex engine. Once inspired and aroused, perhaps you could suggest some steamy scenes in which you and your lover could star in. There is nothing like role play to steam things up! As a precautionary measure, I suggest you refrain from filming your personal porn, instead you both could hold in your minds these sweet memories. The main message here is to be mindful of what you allow to be filmed. Just saying...

Be mindful, whether you are in a long-term relationship or not, communication problems can have an impact on your desire for sex or feelings of sexually arousal. If you are a couple, I suggest you create the time and space for loving communication to resolve areas of misunderstanding. But, a word of caution: we spend so much time trying to resolve disagreements when all we need to do is to "agree to disagree" on some matters. It is impossible to resolve every issue. I've been married and divorced twice, so take it from me, an argument about who "left the toilet seat up", is far too minor for us to allow to escalate. If we do, then boom! Any plans to get some pussy or cock tonight is postponed because somebody is vexed; no fun fucking tonight! Give yourself a break, chill, laugh about some of the disagreements and fuck more often, to create a closer bond between you both. There is nothing like hot, passionate love-making or fucking after an argument; suddenly whose turn it was to wash up becomes null and void!

Here is another juicy pleasure tip. In the tantric traditions, the throat chakra and sex chakra are believed to be intrinsically linked and affect each other. Your voice will help activate your sex chakra to release more sexual energy and more heightened pleasure and powerful orgasm. So, get freaky and open your mouth to say some horny stuff whilst making love. If you're shy, some sexy, sensual moaning will do the trick to give you sweeter, erotic pleasure. Also, together you can spice up your love-making by eating plenty of horny foods, such as peanuts, pumpkin seeds, blueberries, and strawberries, which should be dipped in dark chocolate to increase libido and heighten sexual pleasure. Play around with your favourite toppings or creams to make the experience sweet, slippery and sensual. Use your imagination to determine which of your lover's crevices and curves to apply your toppings and cream. Then enjoy tasting, licking, sucking and eating to your heart's desire. Awaken all your senses to build up to more spark and powerful orgasms. Do a little preparation getting some of these snacks together to make your time awesome.

As an act of foreplay, you can bathe with your lover in preparation in which to indulge each other's crevices and curves. Your pussy has a number of orgasmic areas, including the clitoris and the G-spot. So, if you desire intense 'mind-blowing' orgasms, you could have your lover use their tongue or hand, or both, to stimulate both the clitoris and G-spot simultaneously. Whether you are a heterosexual guy or lesbian woman, be mindful that you are able to help your lover to orgasm. Here's a hot, sexual tip for men who love the pussy - in addition to using your tongue to lick the full contour of her pussy, you will probably need to suck her clitoris. Suction, Suction, Suction! It is like worshipping the pussy!

Equally, as a heterosexual woman or a gay man, ensure you tease your lover's cock before progressing to full-blown penetration. Teasing is done by using your tongue to gently lick your lover's balls; lick the head of his cock, move halfway up the length of his cock, and then proceed to gently take in the full length of the cock in your mouth towards the back of your throat. The 'perineum', which is the area between your pussy and your anus (or your cock and your anus), is known to be a super, orgasmic area, so use your tongue to gently lick this area or use your hand to stroke and transport your lover to dreamy-land.

Tease, tease, tease your lover to enter your wet, moist cave for a treasure hunt or yearn for your juicy, luscious lollipop.

Please note that being a good lover is to ensure that your lover is receiving pleasure from your action. Be present in the moment to your lover's reaction to whatever you are doing. This is also for you even if you have a 'Black Book' full of names indicating your versatility. Previous experience with other lovers is great but less helpful when dealing with a new lover. Each lover is unique; hence you are required to learn that person's pleasure trigger points. Often, there are some concerns around cock or pussy size. With this in mind, it is necessary for lovers to explore more creative ways of satisfying each other. What you might lack in one area, compensate for in others. Use as many of your body parts as you are comfortable with to create an erotic experience with your lover.

Finally, you could experiment with "mirroring and matching" your lover's breathing and body movement. This practice is believed to be able help you to enjoy greater connection with your lover and to heighten sexual pleasure and strength of orgasm. It is simply breathing at a similar pace and creating a dance with your lover's sensual movement.

Scenario

Charles is a 50-year-old Executive in a thriving company. He works long hours and quite often he brings work home, just to keep on top of his duties. He is in a long-term relationship with Judy, a 45-year-old nurse at the local hospital. Charles and Judy started dating 2 years ago and decided to move in together in recent months. Initially, they had a vibrant sex life, however, things began to slow down and they have begun to live more like room-mates. Charles has been having fantasies about fucking an air hostess he met on one of his business trips abroad. He made no attempt to get her details. However, he continues to have thoughts of them being lovers and having steamy sex in every location of the house! She is so darn hot!

Charles is aware that the reason he didn't pursue this air hostess was because he still wants to be with Judy. He recognises that he is not really interested in sleeping with the air hostess, and it was just a fantasy of sleeping with women in uniform, which he has had for some time. Luckily Judy is a nurse and wears uniform. He thinks about exploring the idea of some steamy role play with her. He imagines her dressing up as his night nurse while he acts the sick patient whilst she administers some sexual healing!

Can you relate?

Yes______ No______ Somewhat______

Reflection

Have you been desiring sex? If yes, are you getting enough of the sexual pleasure you really desire? What is it you want to do to spice up your sex life?

BABY, LET'S TRY SOMETHING NEW

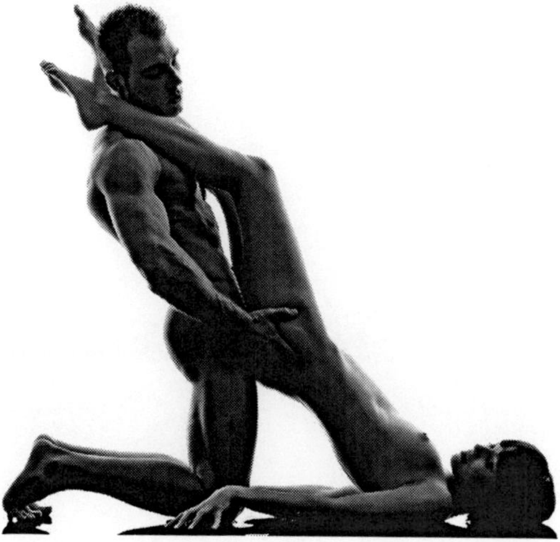

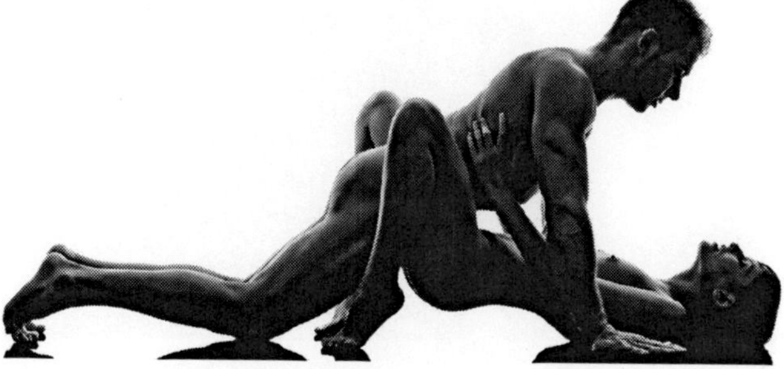

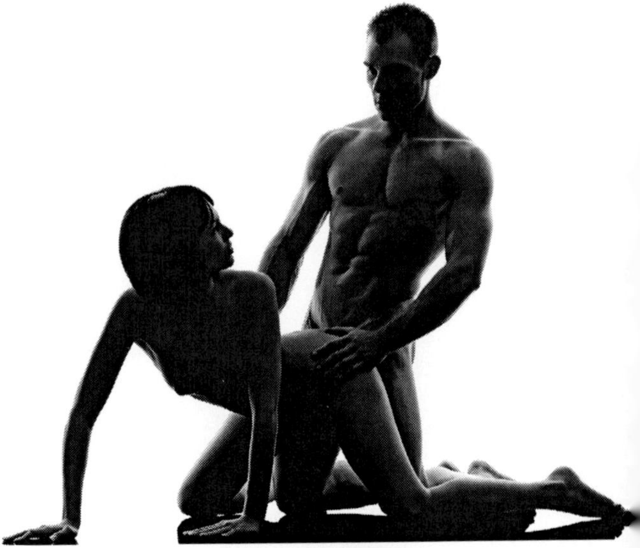

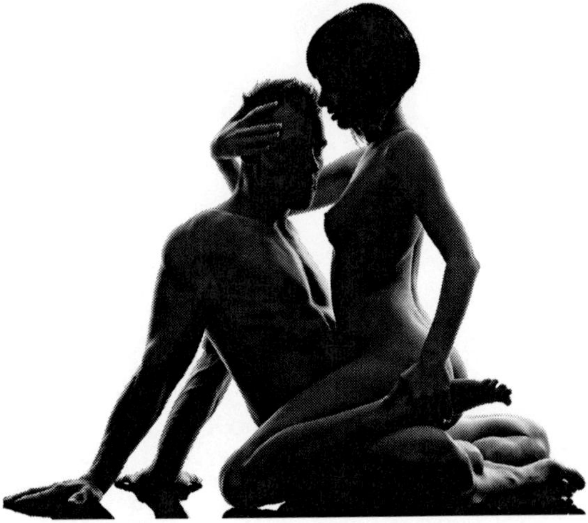

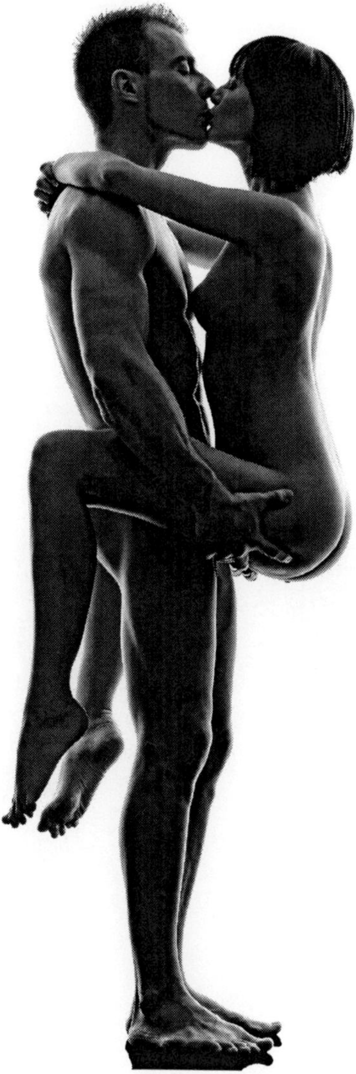

Chapter 3

What Turns You On?

"Guys if her bra matches her panties when you take off her clothes, it wasn't you who decided to have sex!"

– Unknown Author

Do you feel sexy?

Accepting and embracing your sexual story and, more importantly, the image of your body as sexy, can be a key to arousal and the desire for the expression of your sexual self. But do you know what your sexual desires are, physically? Your sexual story and personal desires are important but equally important in your sexual identity, is your body. Determining your sexual story and embracing your sexual self brings confidence and knowledge, equipping you to express the physicality of sex in the most satisfying ways for you.

The media, via books and movies, have conditioned our minds and fed us false definitions of beauty and sexiness. We are fed with perceptions of the ideal body shape and size. Hence, the message is that only the women and men with these preferred bodies have the right to feel sexy and wanted. Well, guess what? News Flash! Most of us, including myself, do not measure up to these ideal body types! So, f**k the media's perception and let's get laid!

If you are definitely overweight and this is impacting on your energy level and ability to move your body in an acrobatic fashion whilst making love, then consider releasing a few pounds without killing yourself in the process. Whilst you probably think that guys go for the slender chick, most men prefer curvy, voluptuous women. This goes for those who are in a same-sex relationship; it might be the case that your lover is and was attracted to you because they love your voluptuous body. Remember also that your unique sexiness is individual. "Beauty is in the eye of the beholder."

There are lots of things we can do to support ourselves to feel sexy in our own skin! Try having long baths with your favourite essential oils, and then just walk around the house butt-naked, especially when you are alone at home. Eventually, you could try walking around naked even when your lover is present, if you are in a relationship. This action of being naked is liberating. Have a go, you deserve it!

I particularly love to dress in clothes that highlight my most favoured body parts. I especially like my breasts and my bum/buttock, so my choice of clothes are usually low cut at the neck and closely-fitted around the hips. I have an array of nicely-fitted lingerie that show off my soft, juicy breasts and voluptuous hips. Hey guys, you can do your thing to enhance how you feel about your body. You don't need to have a six-pack to be sexy. Dress to accentuate your best features and bring on your hunk. We need to take our power back from the media and other parties and redefine the new sexy. Create your individual definition of what you need to do or not do in order to start feeling freaking sexy.

Scenario

Cassidy is a 45-year-old woman with 3 grown children. She has become a bit self-conscious about her sagging breasts and stretch marks, especially whenever she is starting a new romantic relationship. She has struggled for a number of years with the negative perception of her body being unattractive and not sexy. In recent years she has decided that enough is enough, so she embarked on her personal mission to do what she could to enhance her physical appearance of vitality and virility. However, she focused on nurturing her inner beauty and feelings of sexiness. Cassidy started to have regular baths using her favourite essential oils. She would then massage sweet smelling oils into her body and sit peacefully so as to quiet her mind and send messages of love and joy to her inner organs. Cassidy realised that she had been feeling more confident during love-making with her lover and has discovered a zest for life, whilst experiencing heightened pleasure during sexual intercourse

Can you relate?

Yes______ No______ Somewhat______

Reflection

Erection is our physical desire for sex and stems from our own body type and sexual story. Let's focus on your sexual physicality. What body types attract you? What makes you feel attractive? And what do you need in order to feel physically sexual?

SEXINESS BEGINS IN THE MIND...

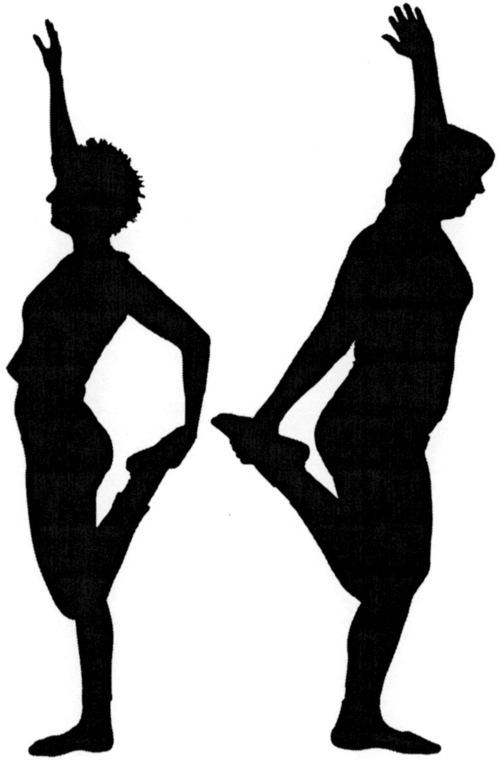

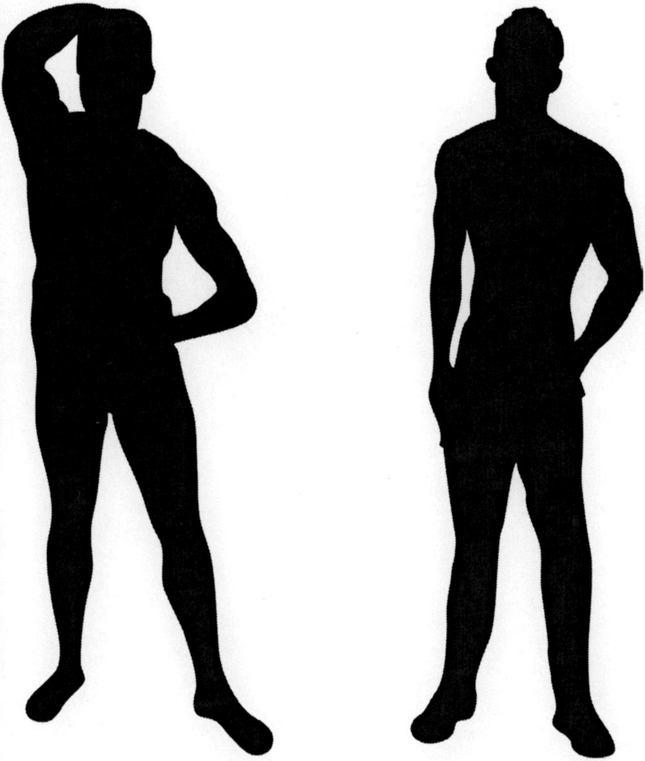

Chapter 4

Can You Go It Alone?

Q: What did the Banana say to the Vibrator?
A: Why are you laughing? I'm the one going to be eaten.

- Author Unknown

Your sexual identity is yours alone, though it may draw others around you. Perhaps your first sexual experience was of self-pleasure or masturbation. On the other hand, perhaps somewhere in your sexual story you have encountered the concept of self-pleasure. The concept of self-pleasure can be formed through watching porn, reading erotica or simply hearing stories of friends reaching the dizzy heights of sexual arousal through masturbation. The beginning of a healthy sexual story should start with a desire, a yearning to explore our bodies, pleasure buttons, crevices and sexual organs. However, this natural urge and desire to finger your pussy and stroke your cock might have been greeted with approval or disapproval by those in your environment. These early responses—positive or negative—will help to shape whether or not you embrace and celebrate your desire for self-pleasure.

Hey you, it is important to explore and connect with your own body in a sensual/sexual way and to understand your likes and dislikes before attempting to share your sweet, sacred beauty with anyone else. How do you expect your lover to automatically know right away how to please you, when you don't even know yourself? You are beautiful in every way and there could never, ever, be any shame in who and what you are. Take your power back from this pleasure-sucking society.

Based on my personal experience and what I have read so far, it is evident that a significant number of us were indirectly taught as children that 'down south' was a no-go zone. We were taught not to even attempt to venture there. I was far into adulthood before I eventually had the guts to look at my beautiful pussy in a mirror. It took me much longer before I started experiencing the sweet pleasure of touching her. I guess, as a guy, you might have a completely different experience of stroking your sweet, delicious, awesome cock, with him being external and right in your face.

Our sexual organs physically represent the possibility and availability for self-pleasure. Though self-pleasure is considered much easier for a man, there are females who are having so much fun with their pussies, wishing they could put their own tongues down south and eat her by themselves. Yes, some women are freaky and living on the edge of a sexual revolution.

There are different means of achieving self-pleasure that include using your finger(s), a dildo, your hand or anything else which is safe that you might think of. You might find reading erotica or viewing films with hot love-making scenes or porn to be helpful in getting you fully aroused. Whatever your method, have fun and get on with it!

Scenario

Tom is a 39-year-old artist, who is in a same-sex relationship with Ron, a 45-year-old teacher. Tom and Ron met a year ago at an Art Exhibition and they instantly knew that they wanted to be together. They enjoy a hot, steamy sex life; however, recently Ron has become a bit concerned as he became aware that Tom still masturbates on a regular basis. Ron was feeling a bit inadequate as he can't understand why Tom would want to continue masturbating if he was fully sexually satisfied.

Ron built up the confidence to talk to Tom about this concern. Tom lovingly explained to Ron that he loves him and he was totally satisfied with their love-making. However, he believes that his personal time of self-pleasure is necessary for him to remain connected with his sexual self. He sees himself as an evolving being, hence his likes, dislikes and idea of pleasure, continues to change as he grows older and therefore his time alone masturbating is mainly for exploration and self-discovery.

Can you relate?

Yes______ No______ Somewhat______

Scenario

Polly is a 47 years old. She has been in a long-term relationship for most of her adult life, and thought that her desire for sexual pleasure and fulfillment was entirely the responsibility of her lover. She didn't see the importance to self-pleasure on her own or during intercourse with her lover, who travelled abroad to work quite often. She was usually sexually frustrated during these temporary separations; however, the latest period was especially frustrating and Polly had no intention of cheating on her lover whilst he was working abroad. Eventually, Polly started to practice self-pleasure and was delighted to enjoy some sweet heaven-bound orgasms. She later communicated her sexual frustration with her lover and they agreed to have sensual, erotic conversations on the phone whilst he was abroad. They also agreed to heighten their phone sex conversation by individually masturbating. Polly and her lover enjoy this so much that they look forward to their phone sex whenever he works abroad.

Can you relate?

Yes______ No______ Somewhat______

Reflection

What has been your experience with self-pleasure? Do you experience desire for self-pleasure? Do you use it to thwart other desires? How is self-pleasure perceived by your family and friends? Is it considered shameful, understandable or desirable?

OH YES, SELF-PLEASURE FEELS AWESOME...

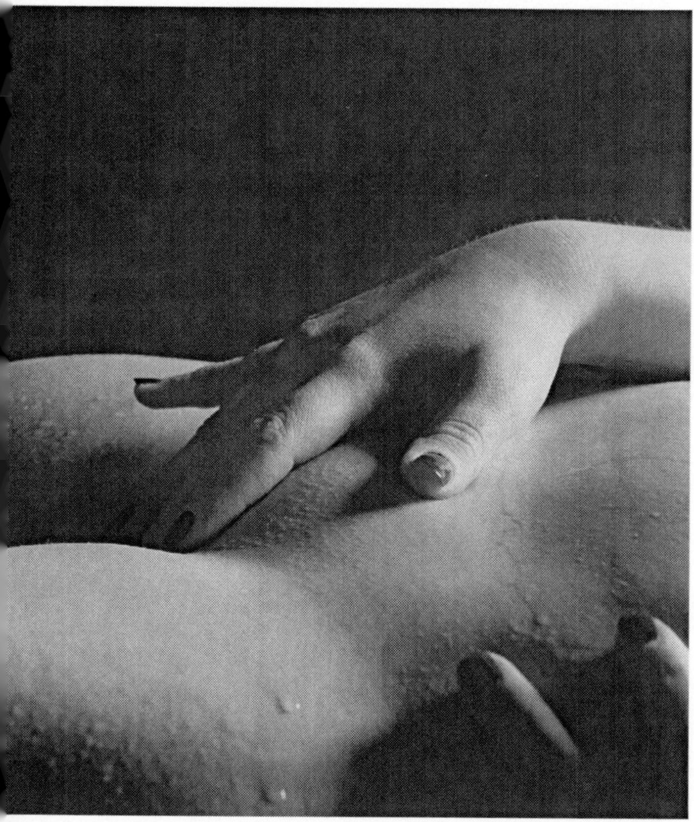

OH MAN, THIS FEELS SO GOOD...

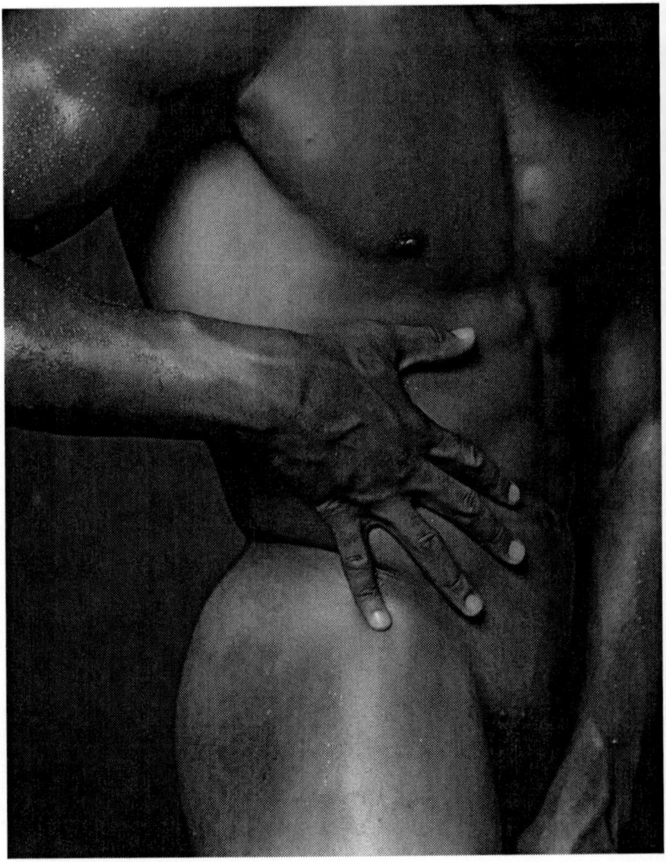

Chapter 5

Dating Your Pussy

Boy: "Want to hear a joke about my dick? Never mind, it's too long."

Girl: "Wanna hear a joke about my pussy? Never mind, you won't get it."

- Author unknown

What is your connection with your vagina?

Whether or not you are in a relationship, regular pussy exploration time equals greater connection with yourself and more erotic sexual satisfaction. This time spent with your pussy is not necessarily for self-pleasure but, more importantly, for self-discovery and connection.

While so much of your physical body plays a part in your sexual experiences, the epitome of your physical sexuality is your vagina (pussy). Your pussy represents the gateway between your sexual mentality and sexual physicality. It is your relationship with this physical part of you that helps develop a deep relationship with your sexual identity.

You receive advances happily but perhaps you do not feel it necessary to initiate your own. Developing a relationship with your sexual self and your pussy specifically will allow you to communicate with yourself and your own needs and desires and, of course, translate them into your sexual life.

An exploration of your relationship with your pussy and how you have and can continue to develop a relationship with this organ, is necessary in order to be true to your sexual self.

Please note that exploring your pussy takes time and patience. You need regular time each week to spend, preferably in front of a mirror where you talk to her, massage her and explore her contours, inside and out. Check out all the pleasure spots and locate your famous G-spot. Regardless of whether you are in a relationship, it is beneficial to know you and become fully sexual with yourself, before you fully share you with someone else. In some cases, you might even need to direct your lover how to please you sexually—where to touch and when.

Some pleasure tips that you might find useful: spend some of the date time with your pussy to flex your pelvic muscles, i.e.: squeeze your pussy muscles as if you are holding in place a small ball. This exercise is meant to tighten the muscles in your pussy so will enhance the contraction and heighten the pleasure for your lover during sexual intercourse, hence more powerful orgasms. This can be done wherever you are; in the office, or in line at the supermarket, among other places. Another pleasure tip is deep belly breathing, which is a relaxation exercise associated with tantric practices that is believed to help you to relax. This practice will in turn clear the pathway to awaken your sexual energy, which can harness greater creativity, productivity and heighten sexual pleasure. This is done by sitting in a comfortable position and relaxing your shoulders. Rest both hands on your abdomen just below your belly button. Breathe in deeply through your nose and into your abdomen so that your belly gently pushes your hands out. Slowly exhale through your nose or mouth allowing your belly to return to normal position. Complete a number of repetitions until you feel relaxed.

Other pleasure tips include giving yourself a full body massage, which is also helpful in connecting with you and circulating your sexual energy around your body. However, be careful with the type of oil you use when massaging your pussy. It is believed that certain oils such as organic coconut oil are best due to its antiseptic healing properties. Finally, talking to or writing letters to and from your pussy, expressing emotions and experiences, is a healing exercise and can aid toward a feeling of connectedness and wellness.

Scenario

Rhonda is a 29-year-old secretary in a large legal firm. She lives on her own in the suburbs however, spends a lot of time clubbing with her friends in the city on weekends. Rhonda occasionally goes on dates; sometimes she sees the same guy but mainly dates different guys.

Rhonda spends most evenings during the week on her own at home. She enjoys long baths with rose petals, lavender and rosemary oils. After these baths, she sits before her mirror and massages her body all over. She gives her pussy a special time of pampering and love. She calls her pussy 'Treasure'. Rhonda always checks in with 'Treasure' about how she is feeling... her likes and dislikes. In one of these conversations, 'Treasure' told Rhonda that she didn't like Jerry, her most recent lover, as he was impatient and wasn't considerate to engage in foreplay but just wanted to jump in and please himself. Rhonda realised that she was also feeling the same way about Jerry for some time, but didn't want to accept it. She had previously shared her concern with Jerry and with no change in his approach, finally decided to stop seeing him.

Can you relate?

Yes______ No______ Somewhat______

Reflection

How do you feel about looking at your pussy? Does this action bring up good or negative feelings for you? Do you believe your pussy is nice looking or ugly? Does it feel awkward or uncomfortable just considering the idea?

CONNECTING WITH YOUR PUSSY IS JUICY...OH YES!!!

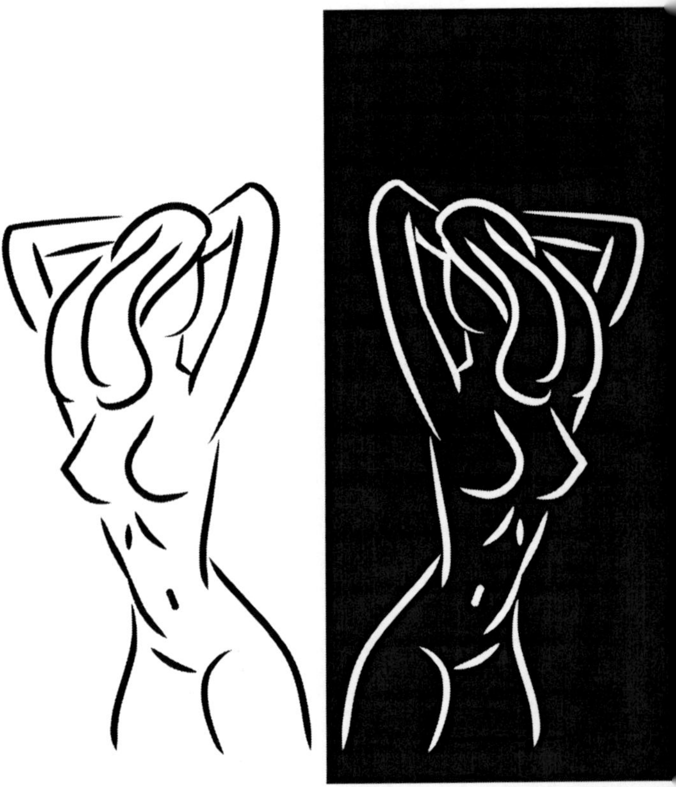

Chapter 6

Cockfoster

"A PENIS is the lightest thing in the world.
Even a thought can raise it."

– Unknown Author

What is your connection with your penis?

While so much of your physical body plays a part in your sexual experiences, the epitome of your physical sexuality is your penis (cock). Your cock is so obviously a part of your physical sexuality but what is less obvious is how it relates to your mental physicality and your sexual self. Unlike a woman's pussy, your cock is very much an external part of your body and is therefore visible to others. Your sexuality is powerful but it is also a deeply connected part of you. You hold a powerful role in sexual interactions, and developing a relationship with your sexual self and your cock specifically, will help you to be in tune with that power.

It is important to explore your relationship with your cock and how it develops and represents your sexual self. You might already have a positive relationship with your cock, which could be as a result of the sexually nurturing environment in which you were raised or experienced as an adult. I am also mindful that it might be the other way round...that you have an unhealthy relationship with your cock due to the negative environment you have experienced and as a result, you might view your cock as a tool of domination to overpower your 'weaker' subjects. I hope you can appreciate what I am about to say and know that I mean it with the best of intentions:

Your cock is a source of pleasure; not an instrument of power and manipulation.

Your lover(s) await the joy and satisfaction that only your cock brings. Pamper him, connect with him, nurture him, feed him and restore his vitality and virility.

Pleasure tips include eating healthy foods, such as pumpkin and sesame seeds, sunflower, strawberries, blueberries...that will nurture your cock, improve sexual agility and increase your sperm count.

Scenario

Barry and Lance are co-workers of a delivery company. Both men spend long days on the street making door-to-door deliveries. They have the opportunity to see numerous hot and sexy women of all shapes and sizes as they drive around each day. Barry and Lance enjoy having fun talking about their fantasies, some of which are not fit for air play or their individual lover's ears. One day Barry shared how he would tie up some women and fuck and whip them mercilessly. This expression was very disturbing for Lance, who was raised in an environment where sex is celebrated and seen as giving mutual pleasure and nurturing to all the people involved. He confronted Barry about his concerns, however, Barry wasn't able to take on board what Lance was saying, as he was convinced that women love to feel pain whilst having sex. Furthermore, if not, they would consider the man inadequate at his job. Both men used humour to melt away the tension, as they agreed to disagree.

Can you relate?

Yes______ No______ Somewhat______

Reflection

How do you see your cock? Is it to give pleasure or to establish power over others? What is your relationship with him? Do you rest him periodically? Keep him healthy?

SEXY IS TAKING THE TIME ALONE TO CONNECT WITH YOUR INNER STRENGTH...

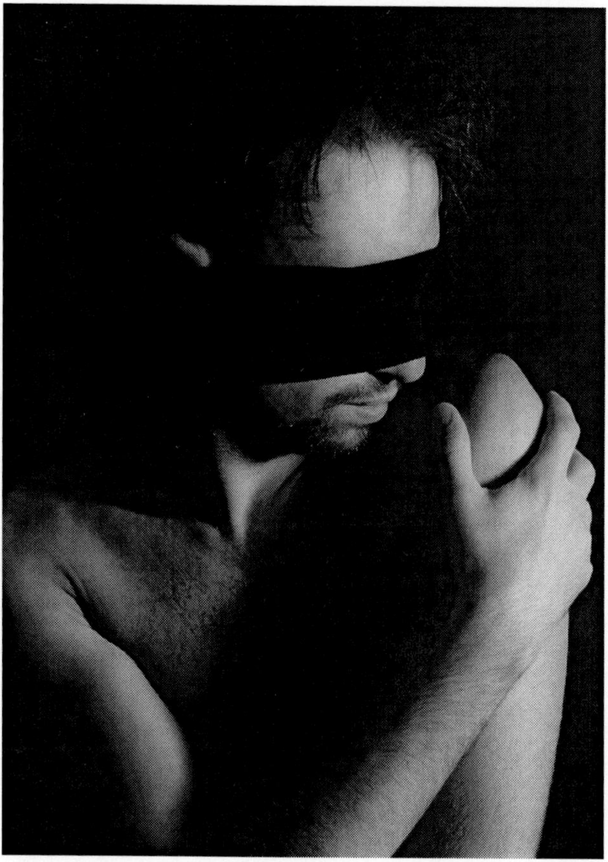

Chapter 7

The Art of Sucking Pussy

Oh, oh, oh Beautiful!

She sits beautifully relaxed on her throne
Like the queen she is
Uniquely Elegant and Poised
Adorned with her dark bushy garment
Oh, oh, oh what beauty!

Her moist, wet, juiciness nurtures her lover
Such a joy to indulge her
Ecstatic pleasure to taste her
Red-hot, bulging with passion
Pulsating to be touched, caressed
Erotic touch-tongue, lips, fingers
Her portal to transport her to the heavenly
Oh, oh, oh what beauty!

– Composed by Jenice Revers

I know that sucking, licking, eating your lover's pussy is such old news. Many ancient societies joyfully indulge in sucking and eating pussy, whether they choose to admit it, that's another point. Still, it is indeed an art of love-making to satisfactorily suck your lover's sweet, juicy pussy. It is an act of worshipping the pussy which can't be accomplished without you perceiving your lover's pussy worthy of great admiration and adoration, mesmerized by its beauty. For us women, it's a delight to be given such great honour and attention. To have your lover's tongue and lips indulge in your moist middle section is heavenly. This is an instant turn-on for us women and can provide all the foreplay necessary for passionate love-making.

The pussy can be perceived as fascinating yet complex structure. I will liken the pussy to a breath-taking, beautiful mansion, situated between two enormous mountains. You will need to take your time to savour, admire, gaze upon, touch her, to fully appreciate her awesomeness. As you wouldn't limit yourself to one small room when exploring an enormous mansion, so you are required to have fun unleashing your tongue along the ridges and contours of this beautiful structure of the pussy. Yes, all the juicy, fleshy, meaty areas. Not forgetting that the top room—the clitoris—loves to be licked and sucked for an awesome orgasm. When stimulated, the clitoris is usually erect like a man's cock, due to the increased blood flow. This erected state of the clitoris allows for your lover to gently grip her with their tongue. Her friend—the G-spot—equally loves the tongue's attention. She is located somewhere towards the lower section of the opening of the pussy.

Be reminded that most women like their pussies to be sucked, eaten, and licked. However, your lover might not like to be fucked in this way. Respect her preference and explore finding other ways of spicing up your love-making.

Simply, the true art of sucking pussy is to suck it, lick it and eat it, just how your lover likes it to be done!

Scenario

Judith is a 20-year-old black woman. She has been in an interracial relationship with Tom, a Caucasian man, for the past 2 years. Judith has had previous lovers; however, she has never experienced such heightened passion and desire for erotic love-making. Judith and Tom do not live together. She continues to live with her family at home. However, Judith visits Tom at his apartment at least twice a week. They usually chat, have a meal together and then watch a movie, yet the evening usually starts or ends with erotic love-making. Judith loves how Tom worships her pussy! Tom enjoys admiring his lover's pussy. He describes the shape, colour and contours of her pussy to her. He says what fascinates him about her pussy. Judith loves these pussy-describing sessions as she can feel her juice starting to flow, getting ready for Tom's tongue, fingers and delicious cock.

Judith is usually taken to heaven when Tom indulges her pussy with his tongue. Tom leaves no crevice or corner of Judith's pussy to be explored. He allows Judith to position her body in various angles over his head. He joyfully rubs his face in her pussy, whilst moaning with great pleasure. He uses his tongue to sweep the full length of her pussy. He dips the tip of his tongue through the opening of her pussy and fiddles around with the G-spot. Tom totally enjoys eating his lover's pussy. He would always have fun with Judith's clitoris, licking, stroking and sucking until he transports his lover to heaven.

Can you relate?

Yes______ No______ Somewhat______

WOW, BABY YOU'RE SO SWEET...

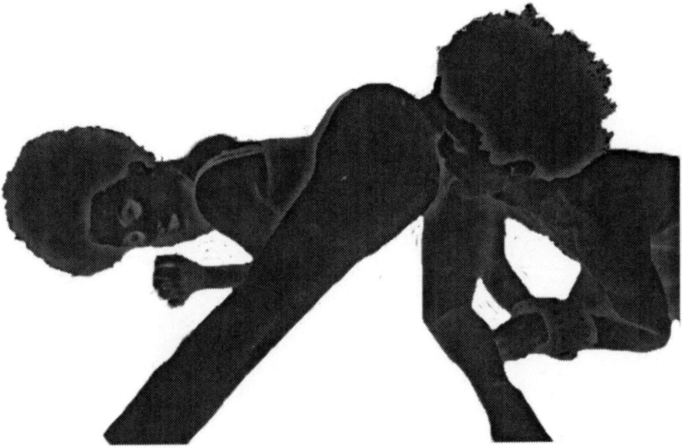

Chapter 8

Black Men and Oral Sex

A daughter asked her mother, "Mom, how do you spell scrotum?"

Her mom replied: "Honey, you should have asked me last night—it was on the tip of my tongue."

– Author unknown

It is one of the sexiest things in the world for your man to text you or call you or to leave a note stating, "I'm going eat all of you!" Girlfriend, this is freaky right! Hey you, I bet your woman's pussy would jump and she would wet her panties in preparation for the erotic love-making that the evening promises. However, it is my understanding that some of our brothers are refusing to "get down" on our sisters, yet they don't mind enjoying the treat of us "licking or sucking their lollipops". Whilst sisters are like "I want you to eat my pussy—and make a meal of it!"

But this is serious though guys...no joke. As black women, we are tired of playing the power games in the bedroom with our men. You are our kings and priests. We love admiring and feeling your strength within and without. We serve you, your children and our society well. So often, we put away our own reservations and surrender to your sexual urges, desires and fantasies—getting down on you is a pleasure for most of us. Likewise, we as black women desire and deserve to be honoured, to be placed on a pedestal inside and outside the bedroom. Some sisters feel forced to take a stance and to go on strike or "lock the pussy shop" or a metaphoric protest signboard saying: "No eating downstairs—no fucking tonight."

I'm an Afro-Caribbean woman, born and raised in the Caribbean. I'm aware of the negative stigma around black men sucking pussy. In my local community, there was the spoken and the unspoken rule that "men don't bow", meaning it was beneath a man to suck or eat a woman's pussy. As a result, most men in my culture either suck pussy but openly deny it or completely refuse his woman this life-giving pleasure. I do understand the pressure black men are likely to experience to fit in with the status quo of what it means to be a "macho man". However, is it manlier to bow to the false pressure, restriction and dictatorship of society's flawed premise or to create your own sexual decisions and unleash your own pleasure between both yourself and your queen? Many of us are doing it anyway so it really is time to "man up". The act of "man up" doesn't necessarily mean you are going to publicise that you suck or eat pussy. The only required adjustment, if any, is for you to free up yourself and give your lover the sweet, delicious experience of sucking her pussy.

Sex is meant to be fun, not a power play or a battle between the sexes. I believe that us as human beings have been given this awesome, live-giving, health enhancing, pleasure-generating ability and we are playing around with it. Let's take our power back. Remove the shame and guilt associated with sex and have some fun in the sack. We all desire and deserve it!

Scenario

Lisa has been with Troy for the past 5 years. They have 2 beautiful children together and they both work to take care of the family. Lisa is somewhat unhappy with her sex life but Troy appears to be fully content and satisfied. Lisa has communicated to Troy that she enjoys sweet hard cock in her pussy but she would also like him to go down on her. Troy has been stalling on the topic and coming up with all kinds of excuses, stating that he has a problem with the smell of pussy. Lisa is offended as she is confident that she keeps her pussy clean and she always has a bath before sleeping with Troy. She doesn't feel that she is getting through to Troy and this frustrates the heck out of her! Getting her sexual needs met in this particular way is very important to her sense of wellness and wellbeing. She has never thought of cheating on Troy before but...

Can you relate?

Yes______ No______ Somewhat______

Scenario

Lenny and Dora have been together for 6 months. Over the past 6 months, Dora has been serving up regular blow-jobs for Lenny but he has been refusing to go down south! Dora wants her pussy to be sucked, however, is afraid to confront Lenny. She is wondering what his refusal is all about?

Can you relate?

Yes______ No______ Somewhat______

Reflection

What's the big deal about "journeying down south" if your lover wants you to? Girlfriends, how are you coping with the fact that your lover is refusing to go down on you?

BABY, I DESIRE TO GIVE YOU TOTAL PLEASURE...

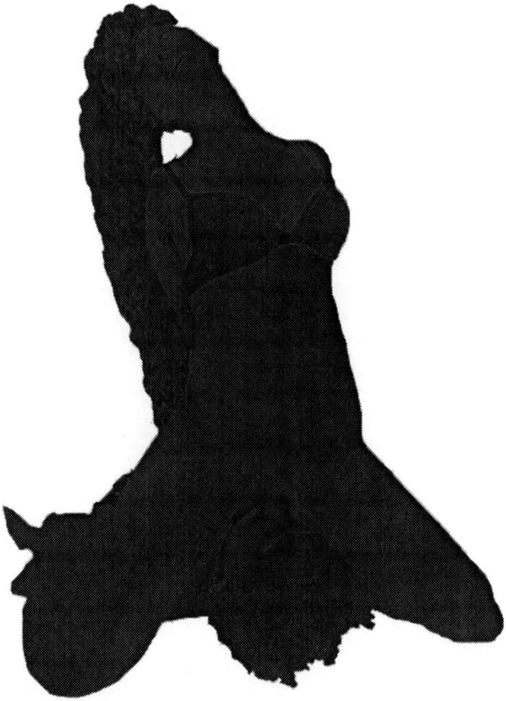

Chapter 9

Fellatio

Awesome Lollipop!

Oh sweet delicious tower of awesomeness
Uniquely shaped and designed
To strike and to conquer
Your prisoners are filled with joy
Hopefully surrendering to your strength.

Your lover melts from your strokes
Long, short strokes
Slowly in and out
Fast throbbing and banging
Yet it soothes the wounds
Heals the soul
Nurtures the bruised
Tantalises the desire to be caressed
Oh, oh, sweet, delicious, juicy lollipop!

– Composed by Jenice Revers

You may or may not be aware of the meaning of 'fellatio' but it is simply "oral stimulation of the penis"; in our case, your lover's sweet, delicious cock. I hope that by this time, there is no need for me to convince you that sucking cock is a normal, juicy and enjoyable part of love-making. If you haven't explored this gem as yet, go ahead and have a ball with it. There is also an art to sucking your lover's cock. The cock is a delicate male organ, especially the tip of the cock and the balls. Don't be fooled by its striking power and visual strength. You are required to handle your lover's cock with gentleness and much care. Allow your lover to direct how gentle or rough you can play with his juicy, delicious cock and balls.

You can worship your lover's cock by allowing yourself to be mesmerised by this beautiful structure of great strength. Be playful and allow the fully erect cock to bounce against your face, across your lips, freely dipping in and out of your mouth. Release your joyful sensual moaning when sucking the cock. Use your tongue to fiddle with your lover's awesome balls. Gently suck on them individually and together to give your lover heightened pleasure. You could suck your lover's cock whilst using your hand to play with his balls, or move between the cock and the balls to spread the pleasure.

Remember, allow your lover to direct you how best to suck his cock for greatest satisfaction. Again, most men like their cocks to be sucked and played with but your lover is a unique individual and therefore this type of love-making may not be to his liking. Don't be turned off, as there as other places on his body you are able to lick or suck that will give him heightened sexual pleasure. Just be willing to explore his body for a more erotic love-making experience.

Scenario

Chris is a 22-year-old male. He has been dating Marjorie who is 25 years old, for the past 3 years. Initially, love-making was routine and somewhat boring. Chris was dissatisfied as Marjorie was shy in expressing herself sexually. She was raised in a conventional family, where sexual expression what inhibited. However, Chris communicated his frustration and they later decided to explore each other's bodies to identify the pleasure spots and eventually they started to enjoy sexual intercourse. They have developed their own style and recipe to sexual pleasure. Chris enjoys it when Marjorie sucks his cock. She usually kneels in front of him and has become such an expert at licking and sucking her lover's cock. Chris also loves it when Marjorie speaks to him during the act of fucking his cock. She would say things such as: "Wow, this is juicy. Give me a taste of your lollipop."

Can you relate?

Yes______   No______   Somewhat______

OH, BABY THIS FEELS SO GOOD...

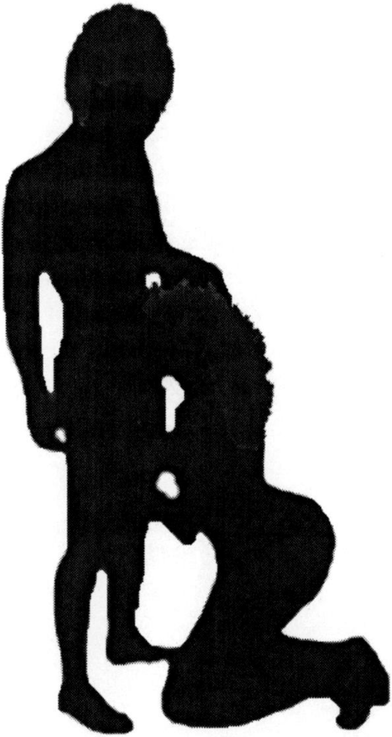

Chapter 10

Full Body Orgasm

ECSTASY

Let go so I can embrace you fully,
Rest your head on my shoulders
Relax your body on mine,
Allow me to taste you,
Nurture you,
Take you to the mountains,
The valley, the planes with me
Soothes you gently
Total ecstatic release.

– Composed by Jenice Revers

Imagine how powerful and intense an orgasm based on genital stimulation is. Well, how amazing and wonderful would it be to experience having similar sexual energy circulated and pulsating all over your body? It is a magical and beautiful experience to behold and to have, something I have seen demonstrated during a tantric massage, while also having experienced it personally.

As mentioned during the introduction to this book, I experienced sexual trauma as a child, which had an impact on my sexual identity and my ability to allow myself to enjoy erotic sex and love-making. I am very sensitive and aware of the struggles some women and men are experiencing with their sexual selves due to sexual trauma they have experienced. However, all is not lost. I have experienced healing through accessing sexual therapy and exploring tantric massage, which includes massaging the yoni (pussy) or cock to enhance stimulation and awaken your sexual energy which is then circulated around the body. This experience is healing for the whole body and soul and specifically re-awakens the numb areas in your pussy or cock.

Tantric massage is an ancient practice that is believed to heal your body, spirit and soul. It boosts full body orgasm whilst harnessing different sexual energy sources within the body and circulates the energy throughout the body. This practice means that you will not be solely dependent on your pussy or cock to experience an orgasm. This massage is both a physical and a sexual experience and is a must try if you want to practise healing and erotic pleasure that result in intense whole body orgasms.

Also, you are able to complete your own massage to reconnect with your body and harness this same sexual energy, whether on your own or with a lover. I am recommending that you plan enough time so you can have a long bath then spend time massaging your body in a slow, tender, sweet manner. Use the type of essential oil that you love as the fragrance will also help to stimulate your sensual nerve. If you have a lover, you could implement this massage as an experience for pure heightened sensation or as a means of foreplay, before enjoying erotic love-making.

Pleasure Tips

In tantric traditions, there is also the method of establishing heart to heart connection with your lover, prior to sexual intercourse, in order to heighten the pleasure and intensity of orgasms. You could achieve heart connection through holding hands and looking into your lover's eyes. This connection also helps you to synchronise your breathing with your lover.

Scenario

Dion is a 35-year-old woman, who was sexually molested as a child. She enjoys a good relationship with men but usually finds it difficult to achieve vaginal orgasm. She would orgasm if she was on top of her lover's hard cock...feeling it slide in and out of her pussy in a rhythmic fashion, whilst he was sucking both her breasts. Dion decided to see a tantric masseur to awaken her sexual energy so she can experience whole body orgasm and multi-orgasms. Her experience of tantric massage has been pleasurable as she enjoys having the inside and outside of her pussy massaged. Dion reported that her massage has helped her to enjoy more pleasurable sensation in her pussy and therefore increasing sexual desire, arousal and intense orgasm.

Can you relate?

Yes______ No______ Somewhat______

Reflection

Are you currently experiencing orgasms on your own and/or during sexual intercourse? Do you desire to experience whole body orgasm? Do you still desire sexual satisfaction? If yes, are you willing to give yourself permission to explore your body and awaken your true sexual self?

OH YES, I FEEL DEEPY CONNECTED TO YOU BODY AND SOUL

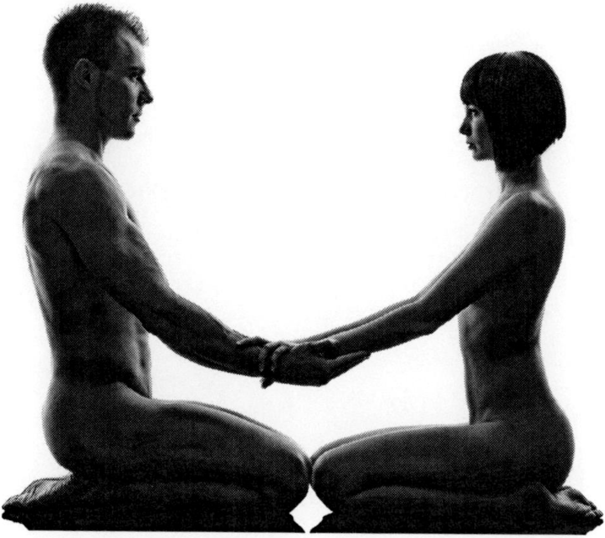

Chapter 11

Monogamy vs Polyamory

After 20 years of sex in the dark, a wife finds out her husband always used a dildo on her!

She said: "Explain the dildo, prick?"

He said: "Explain the kids, bitch?"

– Author unknown

Is having one committed partner more fulfilling than having multiple partners?

Querying which of monogamy or polyamory is more beneficial is a value-laden question. The answer I assume is down to individual taste, personality type, preference, lifestyle and the belief system/values of 'should' and 'should-not' ascribed to. At the end of the day, it's about what makes you happy, provided you are upfront and honest with your lover and they are in agreement with it. Research concludes that sexual pleasure releases a complex set of hormonal responses in the brain that the body uses for supporting physical, emotional, and mental health. These chemicals include serotonin, ocytocin, dopamine and endorphins. However, please note that the benefits received from the release of these chemicals are not limited to people in monogamous relationships but to everyone who engages in sexual intercourse. Serotonin is referred to as the "feel good hormone". It helps people to feel relaxed, peaceful, happy and contented. Oxytocin is also known as the "cuddle hormone" because it causes people to form bonds. It is stimulated in the body through touch and sexual orgasm. Dopamine is a neurotransmitter that generates feelings of bliss. Endorphins are feel-good chemicals produced in the brain. Some of these chemicals lower stress, improve immune system functions, induce a general sense of well-being, help us to relax and increase levels of confidence.

I believe that our society has conditioned,

especially women, to believe that we can only be happy and satisfied in a committed relationship with one lover. Some would argue that a woman's natural physical and emotional make-up (having an internal vagina that causes her to take in), determine that she is more likely to form emotional attachment and experience greater fulfilment, by being in one committed relationship.

There is also research to support the theory that men are better able to enjoy and appreciate the physicality of sexual intercourse without becoming emotionally attached with the women or men they sleep with. Based on this premise, it could follow that men are more likely to be happier than women if they choose to have relationships with more than one lover. I'm sensitive to the physical/emotional make-up of us women but personally, I partly agree with the whole "women are naturally more emotional and are more likely to form emotional attachment with each sexual encounter" argument. I strongly believe that we as women were raised to be "good girls" and that we should find a man and get married, have children and take care of the home and everybody else, except our own needs. As a woman, I dare you to express your needs for a more intense sexual experience or desire to explore your fantasy or lifestyle of sleeping with more than one man. I believe some women truly desire this freedom, especially during different periods of their lives. Yet our pleasure-sucking society attempts to dump on them restrictive ideologies and condemnation for having these 'unmentionable' desires.

I recently saw a post on Facebook and felt compelled to respond to it, due to the derogatory nature of the assumption. Here we go:

Facebook Post

"How many females can honestly say you have only been with one man in 2015?"

My Response

Why does how many men a woman has been with, within a year matter? This is a value judgement that we all must stop as people. It does impact on some women who haven't yet realised that our value is NEVER defined by our experience...we are all awesome: period. Back to the original point, none of us know the reason why any woman has been with one or a number of men this year. It might be that she adores celebrating her sexuality in that way and that's OK or that she has been played by a number of brothers, even though she desperately wants to settle down?

Yes, indeed, you might desire or prefer a monogamous relationship and that's OK. It is important that you be true to yourself, therefore, wait for the type of relationship you want. However, when you are in such a relationship, make full use of it and explore and unleash your sexual urges, desires and passion. Enjoy yourself being sexually free with your lover. At the same time, there are some women and men, who are confident and are sexually versatile and so are equally able to enjoy the benefits of a monogamous or a polyamorous relationship. Whether in a monogamous or polyamorous relationship, you are able to enjoy the pleasure of sex and I strongly believe that's OK too!

Guys, kings and priests, please don't take what I am going to say next as an offence or as any power game. However, I believe that anything a man can do (sexually and emotionally), a woman can do too, if left alone to explore her natural curiosity with sex and her sexuality. Yes, some women do have fun sleeping with different lovers also!

Finally, I do believe that as human beings, we are able to enjoy beautiful and fulfilling sexual relationships with one lover or with multiple lovers, without any short-term or long-term emotional repercussions. It is our society that has conditioned, especially women, to not fully explore our sexual urges and desires. This nature vs nurture argument will continue but no research can speak for everyone; it is an assumption based on the general responses given to a particular stimulus. We are unique, so follow your heart and free yourself from mental slavery.

Scenario

Susan is 35 years old and an independent career woman who lives in a major city. She has had polyamorous relationships and has enjoyed them all. She has beautiful memories of the erotic love-making with her lovers and is pleased that her relationships all ended with all parties on good speaking terms. She values her sexual health, so ensured she used condoms during each sexual experience.

Lately, Susan's sexual energy has changed and she is feeling a new excitement to date only one man and continue to enjoy her f**k experience. Susan is now seeing Paul, however, she has other guys who are asking her out but she is now committed to having a monogamous relationship at this period of her life, whilst having fun flying on her erotic high.

Can you relate?

Yes______ No______ Somewhat______

Scenario

Nadine is a 40-year-old free-spirited woman. She has been dating Paul for the past 18 months. She was clear in communication with Paul from the beginning of their relationship, that she was happy with an open relationship in that they could see each other regularly on a weekly basis, sleep together, eat out and even travel together. However, she was happy seeing both men and women and over the past 18 months whilst with Paul, she has dated a few women and continues to see at least one of them on a regular basis. Paul is aware of this and continues to be happy with their relationship arrangement.

Can you relate?

Yes______ No______ Somewhat______

Scenario

Sally is a 45-year-old single woman. She has been in long-term relationships and has thoroughly enjoyed them. However, she is single at this stage of her life and just wants to have some fun exploring sex and her sexuality. She has a quest to enjoy herself, having lovers from various cultural backgrounds. Sally especially would like lovers from Spanish, Italian, British, American, Canadian, Caribbean, African, Asian, and Middle Eastern backgrounds. She travels a lot for work across America and Europe and likes to explore the city night life after a busy day working.

Sally feels well sustained and nurtured by this lifestyle. As a sexually empowered woman, she exercises her choice about which man to sleep with or who to go out with socially. She doesn't feel pressured to fuck any man due to his position of power or influence over her life. Her experience of fucking her different lovers is just so alluring and delicious. Sally is having a lot of fun with her chosen lifestyle.

Can you relate?

Yes______ No______ Somewhat_____

Reflection

What are your thoughts on the subject of monogamy vs polyamory? Do you feel able to freely act on your desire for polyamorous relationships, if this is what you want?

IT'S YOUR CHOICE TO MAKE...

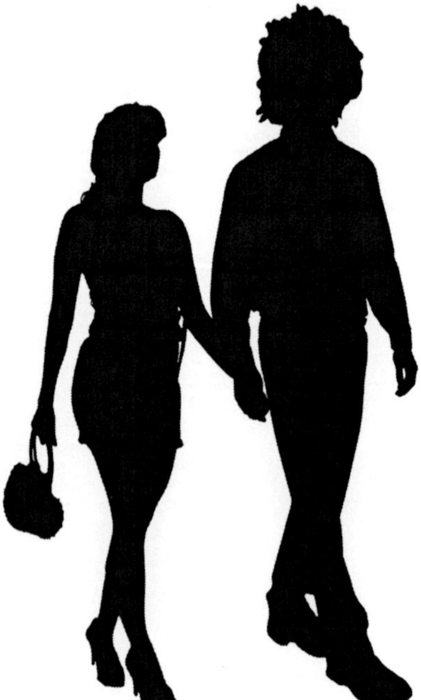

MONOGAMY

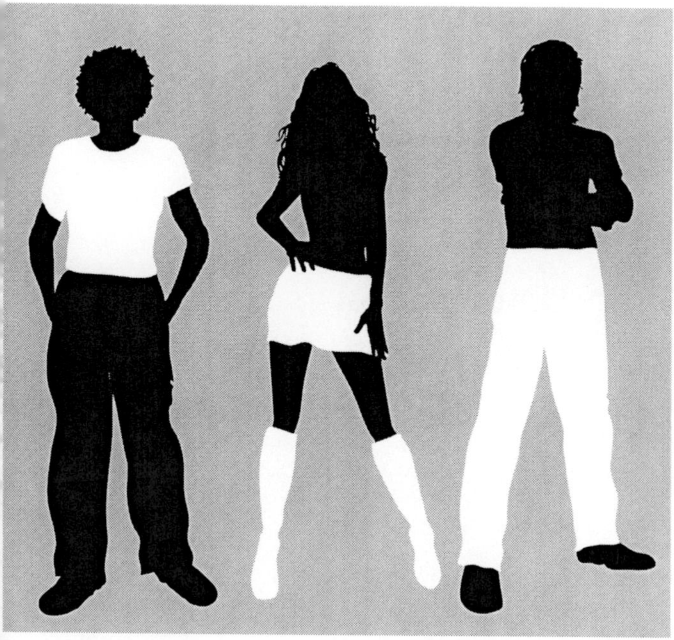

VS POLYAMORY

Chapter 12

Heterosexual vs Same-Sex Relationship

“Love will show you the way home.”

- Composed by Jenice Revers

As I ponder this issue of heterosexual vs same-sex relationship, a flood of questions emerge. Why does one's relationship or sexual preference matter? Why is this an issue that others feel they need to express an opinion about? ? Isn't there a free option for each adult? Doesn't each consenting adult have a right to decide their sexuality? Why is this society so ingrained in intolerance around differences? Why do we aim to make ourselves right and other people so wrong, by virtue of exercising their right to choose who they want to sleep with?

Provided sexual intercourse is between consenting adults, what do I care about who is sleeping with whom?

I have friends who are happy and satisfied in their heterosexual relationships and others in same-sex couplings, who are equally happy and content in their relationship. Based on my previous religious beliefs, I would have negatively judged people who were in same-sex relationship. However, I feel that my evolution has brought me to an enlightened position where I am tolerant of people and their right to choose what they believe, how they act and the lifestyle they embrace. I believe this is an individual choice and nobody has the right to enforce their belief on another person. Your beliefs are not right and other people's beliefs are not wrong. They are all called beliefs for a reason because they are just that and not 'truth'. What is the standard or measuring stick for 'truth'? It is all perception. We live and experience this world based on our individual perception. Allow people to live their lives how they choose, provided it has no effect on your life.

We live in a society that believes heterosexual relationships are the ideal. They use the 'nature' argument to support this by stating that same-sex relationships are not consistent with nature, as the couple cannot procreate together. I do agree that procreation is integral to the continuation of our human lives. However, we do not all need to procreate for humanity to evolve. Even some heterosexual couples are exercising their choice whether or not they want to contribute to procreation. Is it our main purpose on earth to procreate? Some people will say 'yes' and their life choices will reflect this, while others will say 'no' and their life will be consistent with their responses.

I don't believe that our purpose here on earth is communal and that we are all supposed to be doing the same thing. Let your heart be your guide. Your heart, if not contaminated by other people's views, won't lie. At the end of the day, what I am saying is you are free to make your own decision about your life. I believe that you are not here to suffer but to create, prosper and have fun loving yourself and others. I am aware that even my understanding is limited, so follow your heart's directions. Live your life how you choose and love who you choose and let the rest of us suck it up if we don't like it!

Scenario

Marlon is 44 years old and has been married and divorced twice. All his life he had only been attracted to women. However, since his 44th birthday, he has been having new emerging erotic feelings towards other men. Marlon wants to explore these new feelings, so he decided to take matters into his own hands and browsed the internet for gay bars in London. He went on his night out on the town by himself and before the night was over he kissed a man for the first time and he liked it. Marlon didn't get the full experience on his first night out, yet he is committed to following this new desire for same-sex intercourse.

Can you relate?

Yes______ **No**______ **Somewhat**______

Reflection

Do you feel that you are currently in a relationship that reflects your true sexual preferences or desires? If not, are you empowered to act consistent with your true inner erotic desire?

LOVE IS YOUR COMMON GROUND...

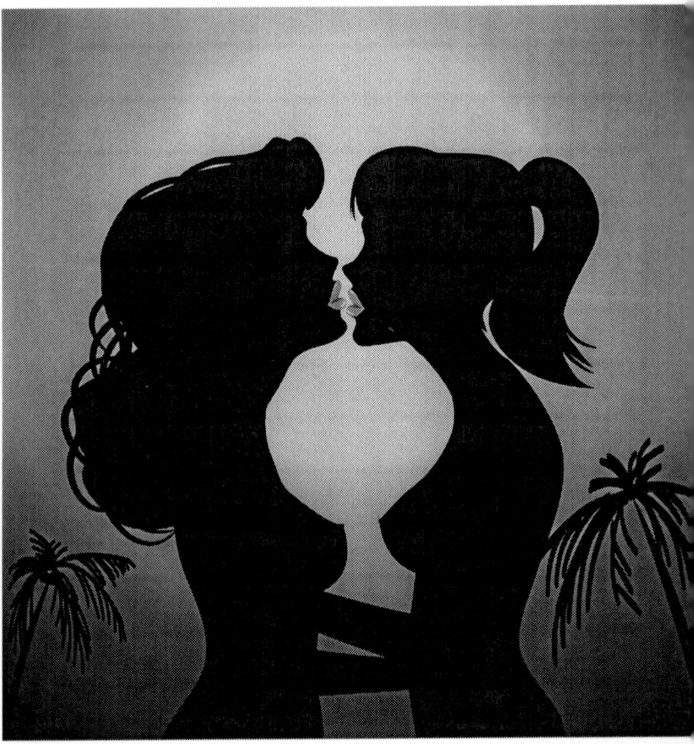

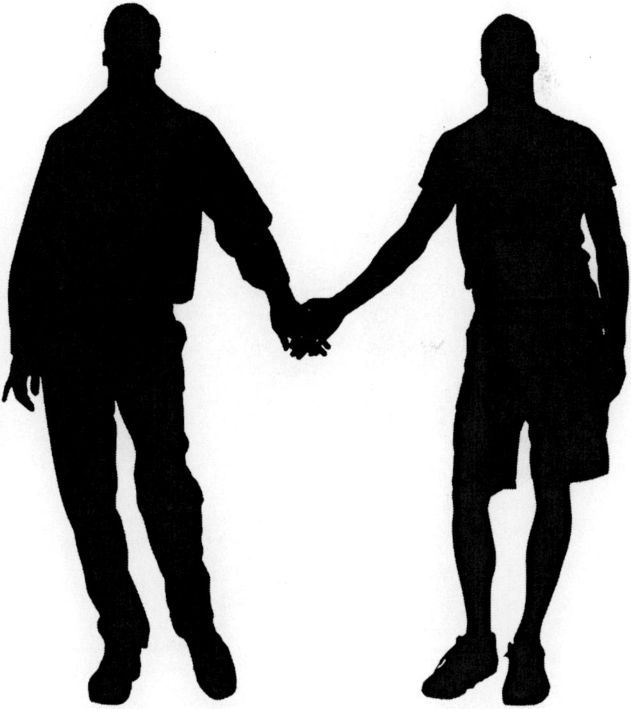

SAME SEX RELATIONSHIP

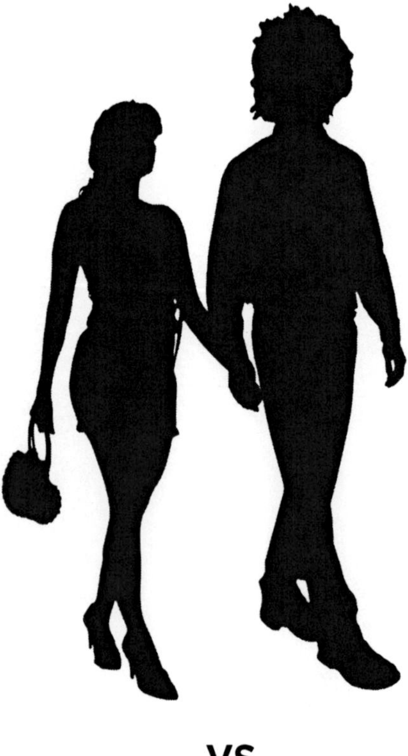

VS

HETEROSEXUAL

Chapter 13

Good Girl vs Bad Girl Syndrome

"Does my sexiness upset you?
Does it come as a surprise?
That I dance like I've got diamonds
At the meeting of my thighs?"

– Maya Angelou

There is a saying: "Good girls go to heaven whilst bad girls go everywhere!" And, I will add, have all the fun. I believe this "good girl vs bad girl syndrome" is a value judgement instilled in us since childhood. However, our adherence to this as grown women is causing us to be sexually unsatisfied, unfulfilled and sometimes miserable. The time has come for us to take control of our power and choose how we express our own sexuality.

Woman! Every part of you is beautiful. Don't allow society, religion, men or other women to cause you to feel dirty due to your desire to dress sexy and celebrate your sensuality. Instead, we as a society are required to exercise tolerance, knowing that a woman's decision to embrace and celebrate her sexuality/sensuality via her style of dress or otherwise, is hers only and should be respected. As I completed my research for this book, I was even more awakened to the double standards in our society. We have a society that celebrates contestants wearing swimwear in Beauty Pageants, erotic expressions such as belly dancing and carnival soca groove, whilst condemning images of Beyoncé, Rihanna and gyrating in dancehall as lewd and sleazy! In the media, there are constant attacks on the sexy images of women.

Some people go as far as to say that women who choose to dress sexy have lost their dignity and their position as role-models for other women, children and their homes. There are others who suggest that we as women can't be sexy and smart, intelligent, strong, and independent. Some women in the spotlight are perceived as being used for economic reasons to sell music, cars etc. This view is presented as if we have no choice but to flaunt our assets (beautiful bodies) for economic reasons. Isn't it the same way as others capitalise on their talents of acting, singing, accounting, nursing, teaching? Get a life, people. Most of these women posing on a car or in music videos are wearing swimsuits or other skimpy clothing similar to our famous beauty pageant contestants. Where is the difference?

In order to maintain human dignity, I sincerely believe that instead, we as a society need to focus on teaching our boys and men boundaries, self-control and respect for other people's bodies—exposed or unexposed. Hey, guys, I am well aware that research supports that you are 'visual', meaning that you are sexually stimulated by what you see. However, your natural urges or inclinations are not an excuse for you not exercising self-control. There are times when we women see a 'fine-looking' guy with bulging muscles above and down below and we look on lustfully and sometimes tell our girlfriends about this luscious sight. But how often do you hear of a woman walking up to a man on the street and grabbing a hold of his cock (as tempting as that is)? We are 'visual' beings too! If you didn't know, now I'm telling you that we sometimes look at you and lust about feeling your strength and tasting you, also.

Some women may agree with dressing sexy,

however, they go further to create another box about what is sexy vs sleazy. Isn't this based on individual taste and value system? Why should we continue to expect other people to live their lives based on our personal experiences, values and preferences? As people—I have said this before but I will repeat it again—we are socialised to fear and to be intolerant of difference. We appear to gain a sense of superiority in making other people wrong, especially about their sexuality.

Views such as women who gyrate or move their hips in a sensual manner are lewd and sleazy, need to be challenged. For some people, these movements are too sexual in nature and as a society, some of us are so afraid of anything sexual. Some people are of the volition that this type of disgraceful action should be banned to the dark dungeon of the bedroom.

I'm personally aware of women in steady relationships who are sexually inhibited. They continue to behave like a "good girl" as that was the standard necessary to attract the man of their dreams. However, if you are such a woman, you might be surprised to know if you already not aware, that most men would like you to behave like a lady in public and a pole-dancer, or a stripper in the bedroom. It's all about your ability to play many roles. You are already juggling many balls and wearing many heads in your life. We juggle many roles, parts and characters in the office, as a parent, as a friend etc. So get on with it and put your fuck hat on. Enjoy your life!

As a result of my recent interest in Tantric and other holistic practices, I became aware of the importance of losing ourselves in the pleasure of movements. Sexual/sensual movements contribute to our general feelings of wellness and wellbeing. It is also believed to awaken and help to circulate our sexual energy around our bodies. In the holistic sector, we are referred to as a top-heavy society (intellectually-focused), as we spend a lot of time in our heads. We are not spending enough time living in our bodies, connecting with the essence of what it means to be fully human and experiencing the moment. Regular dance and movements are considered to be essential to physical, emotional, and spiritual wellbeing for both men and women. Sensual dance and movements, which includes moving the pelvic regions, are especially healing for women as it focuses on flourishing our feminine qualities.

Again, I say, take your power back from this pleasure-sucking society which wants to dictate the intimate details of how each of us lives our life. Work, work, work, productivity, results, burn-out.... We all need regular fuck breaks, time to dance, move and connect with the true essence of life itself. We have somewhat lost what it means to be human beings. We fail to 'be' and are always 'doing'. Let's start moving our bodies more, especially our pelvic region—this is deliciously sweet, sensual and life-giving.

Scenario

Shanika loves to dress trendy and sexy! Her outfits are usually deep cut at the neckline and closely-fitted around the hips. Shanika feels her choice of fashion is her truest self- expression and she loves it. She regularly goes out partying with her friends, however, some people appear to be disturbed by her style of dressing and how she is moving her body in a sensual manner. She notices the constant stares of disgust, especially from other women, which she finds somewhat disturbing, despite her being a confident person. She sometimes feels that she would want to ask what are they staring at but she resists getting into a confrontation over what is her personal choice of dress.

Can you relate?

Yes______ No______ Somewhat______

Scenario

Lora is a middle-aged woman who is an Executive in an Accountancy Firm. Most of her colleagues are male and they wear mainly black or grey suits to the office. Lora, however, loves to wear bright coloured suits, which she finds sexy. Her shirts usually have deep cut necklines and her pants are closely-fitted at the hips. Recently, Lora was approached by one of her senior executives who implied that she was causing distraction in the office. She was a bit annoyed, as there are a number of male colleagues who wear tightly-fitted trousers that have their cock and balls almost plucking out through their zippers. Lora thinks, 'What's this all about?'

Can you relate?

Yes______ No______ Somewhat______

Reflection

What is your definition of being sexy and sensual? How comfortable are you to express yourself as a sexual/ sensual being? Are you fully embracing your sensual expressions?

DEFINE YOUR OWN SEXY...

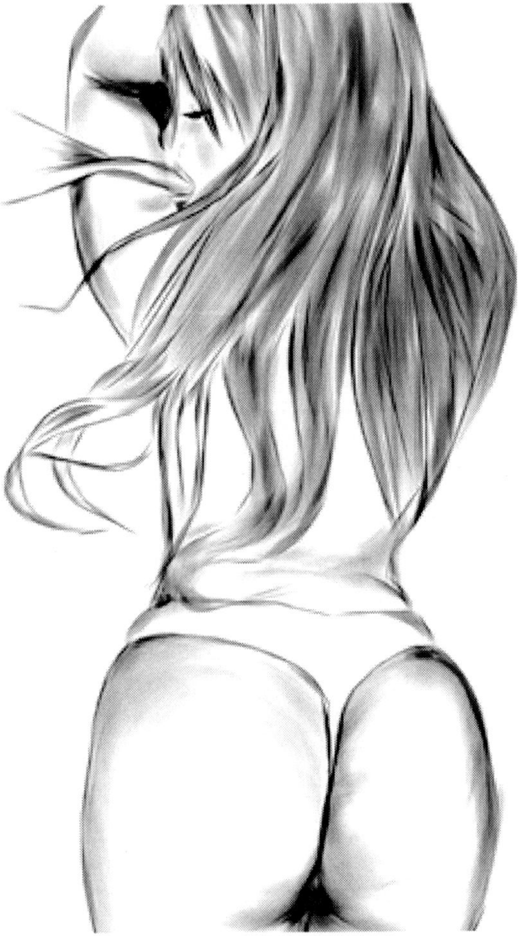

Chapter 14

Putting Your Wish List in Action

FANTASY

Fascinating blissfulness
Appealing lust
Never-ending curiosity
Thrill of the unknown
Abounding sweetness
Seductive juice
Yielding desires

– Composed by Jenice Revers

Are you satisfied with it? You are in tune with your sexual self. You have faced your sexual experiences and are mindful of how these have shaped your sexual identity. You have developed a relationship with your physical sexuality and your sexual organs, and you know what you want and what makes you feel your most empowered, sexual self. But will you communicate it to others? Will you get what you want from your sexual experiences?

No matter how confident we feel, it can be nerve-wracking to own up to our sexual fantasies. You know them yourself, but it can be difficult to open yourself up to another person. And then there are the other questions: Is your lover capable of fulfilling your sexual fantasies? What if it does not live up to your fantasy? What if you chicken out? There are so many 'what ifs' but we must allow ourselves to fantasize, to want our fantasies, and to communicate them. We must also allow ourselves to explore our fantasies in order to be truly fulfilled.

I am aware that many women and men would not dare to ask for their fantasies to be met due to limiting beliefs based on society's Shoulds and Should Nots.

The term 'Should' is disempowering, although if replaced with 'could' indicates a choice, rather than a rule.

Replaced with: "I could be lady-like. I could make an advance for sex." (A choice)

Go ahead and write down your own limiting Should and Should Not beliefs around sex and replace should and should not with 'could'. OMG! This feels freaking empowering; yes, choices usually give you that powerful feeling.

My aim is to encourage you to explore how you manifest your sexuality in your communication. It is my hope to have you confidently speaking about sex and engaging in the sex-talk you find pleasurable. It is one thing to be mindful of your own sexual self, and it is important to develop the confidence to embrace it wholeheartedly. However, what takes confidence is the extra step to empowerment and the ability to communicate this confidence with others.

A group of women met in a workshop to discuss what they really wanted. Below is the list of wishes they come up with:

- Someone to have rough sex with me
- Orgy with men and women
- To be blindfolded whilst having sex
- Demand sex from a stranger
- Submission
- Eating pussy
- A man to watch me make a woman cum
- An audience whilst having sex
- Spend a whole day having sex
- Seeing live porn together with my partner
- Sexual adventures
- Orgy party
- Swingers party
- Sex with ladies
- Threesome

Pleasure Tips

First, you could start by exploring with your lover the idea of trying out some of your fantasies that do not include a third party. Of course, this would need to be something your lover feels comfortable with as we would commonly say, "two can't walk together, unless they agree". Later, when you are more confident, you could explore the possibility of trying others. For example, if you have a fantasy of having sex with men or women in uniforms, it may be a good idea to buy some props, such as fireman helmet or sailor's cap, police officer's badge or whistle, nurse's cap, air hostess' accessories, or the full set of uniform, if you are able to afford it, so that your lover can dress the part. As suggested earlier, you may consider watching porn together and then suggest that you act out your own porn movie. Give yourselves names for each leading actor/actress and decide the storyline you will be role-playing. If you are single and dating, you can get in on the action with your date, however, you just might need a bit more preparation to make it happen.

If you are shy and struggling to communicate your fantasies with your lover, try writing it on paper first and then practice saying it out loud in front of the mirror. Practice, practice, practice, until you gain your confidence. You could write your lover a note and leave it for them to see. You could start a hypothetical conversation around, "Suppose someone you were with wanted to do a threesome, how would you view it?" Or,

"How would you feel if I wanted you to handcuff and fuck me?" If you don't ask, you might never know if you could have your fantasies fulfilled. Your lover might be ready for the fun and exploration.

Just a bit of caution here; I am aware that the porn industry has created unrealistic fantasies around sex, especially for men. Guys, please be mindful that porn is a paid professional performance of a fantasy scenario, so don't use it as your education. Most women are not as orgasmic as portrayed in porn films. Some women don't like to be fucked at high speed for long periods. Neither do most men have such lengthy 10-inch cocks. The scenarios in porn are extreme; hence it is sometimes unrealistic to expect your lover to fulfil all the desires that have been awakened. However, don't be discouraged as you might never know, your lover might be as kinky as you are. He or she might be just waiting for you to mention it. There are porn scenes where one woman is being fucked in the mouth, pussy and ass at the same time. Anal sex is quite common in porn films. Still, I am quite aware that there are various sexual fantasies beyond the scope of what is viewed in porn films. Remember, sex should be consensual, whether or not you are in a long-term relationship. The act should be equally desirable and pleasurable for your lover. You have a right to refuse to engage in any act that makes you feel uncomfortable or may harm you in any way.

I must interject that there is a risk that you might share your sexual fantasy with your lover and they reject it for whatever reason. You might decide that it is no big deal, so you can happily continue your relationship. However, you might also decide that to fulfil this fantasy is very important to your overall sexual fulfilment and satisfaction. As a result, you are faced with the decision of your personal happiness or the continuance of this relationship. It might be a big decision for you to make, but hey you deserve to be happy so you will be required to make some tough decisions. These decisions are necessary and fulfilling this fantasy may be crucial to your happiness. I am aware that there is a need to compromise for any relationship to succeed but the question is, how much can anyone be expected to compromise? I certainly don't believe in compromising your own happiness. The decision is yours whether to stay or to leave this relationship. Take your power back and choose!

Resist from ridiculing your lover, should they communicate their desire for a sexual act that doesn't interest you. Instead, you could say: "That's interesting. I've not thought about that before and am not sure how I feel about it. Can we check in with this idea a bit later?" It is common for some lovers in short-term and long-term relationships to have two separate sex lives. One where they engage in the 'normal' routine sex with their steady lover and another where they either watch porn, or sleep with a prostitute, or have a lover or lovers on the side. The decision is yours if you want to continue to live in misalignment to your true self. FREEDOM is living in your truth! One thing I am very sure of is that a lot more fucking can take place and fantasies fulfilled within your current relationship, whether short-term, long-term or dating.

Scenario

Dawn is 46 years old, has been married to Stephen for the past 13 years and they have two lovely children aged 9 and 11 years. They are both Christian, therefore Dawn assumed that sex during their marriage was going to be the "biblical way" (that is vaginal). However, soon after her marriage to Stephen, she was distraught to find out that he expected both vaginal and anal sex. Dawn had given in because she wanted Stephen to be happy and to save her marriage but she has been hurting both physically and emotionally over the past 13 years. Stephen is aware of her discomfort and pain during anal sex, yet he continues to demand to have his desires met. Dawn is considering ending her marriage, as she believes that Stephen fails to consider her physical and emotional welfare.

Can you relate?

Yes______ No______ Somewhat______

Scenario

Cassandra and Phillip have been happily married for the past 15 years and they have 3 beautiful children. They continue to enjoy an active, erotic sex life. Cassandra and Phillip are very open in sharing their fantasies with each other and are willing to explore each one of them, after much discussion. They have both enjoyed oral, vaginal and anal sex and they have done a lot of role-playing, which includes dressing up as different characters that causes sexual arousal for each of them.

Can you relate?

Yes______ No______ Somewhat______

Reflection

Is there something you desire sexually that you are able to say explicitly, or do you struggle to talk 'dirty'? What are your sexual fantasies and what is your wish list? How can you act on them with your partner or alone?

OH YES, BABY LET'S GET NAUGHTY TONIGHT!!! I WANT US TO...

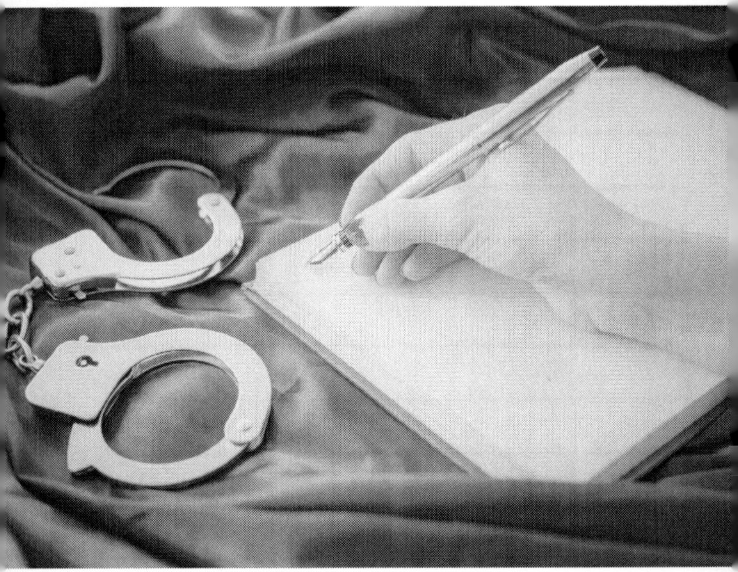

Final Word from the Author

Throughout this book, we have explored the ideas of both natural and learned sexual identities and how they combine to make your own unique sexual identity. We have also explored how mental and physical sexualities and desires combine to create your sexual self and how previous and current experiences are all important factors in your sex story.

Empowered with this knowledge and self-reflection, you hold all of the tools to empower your own sexuality and sexual experience. Remain mindful of your body, your mind, and yourself. You shape your sex story with your experiences and your reaction to them. You shape your sexual experiences through your own confidence and communication. You are in charge of your sex story now.

You have a beautiful, sacred treasure in the form of your pussy or cock, ready to be explored and to enjoy all of the intense pleasure of passion, desire and orgasm. So, what are you waiting for! Take your power back and start enjoying your life and LET'S GET LAID!

OH YES, BABY
LET'S GET LAID...

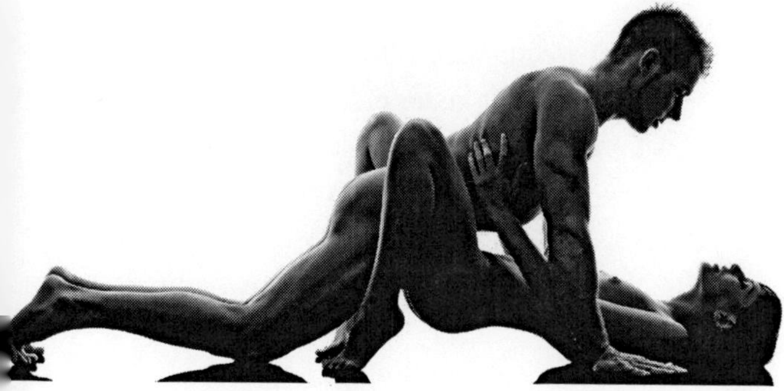

PULSATING DESIRES

Indulge your burning passion,
Caress her, soothe her,
Look into your tantalizing eyes,
Dazzled by the heat of erotic love!

Captivate me with your pulsating desires!
Wet, soft kisses of lusciousness
Consumed with your moans of ecstasy
Bodies and hearts eclipse
Desires are quenched and the weaves of passion cease.

– Composed by Jenice Revers

PULSATING...PULSATING...
PULSATING

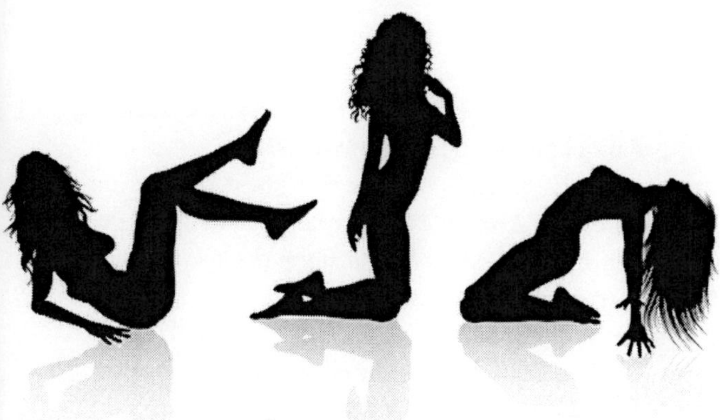

Author's Biography

Jenice Revers is an empowerment specialist. Her passion for helping and healing has led her to many roles, including teacher, counsellor, social worker, author, speaker and mentor. She has been a social worker and an independent advisor to the Family Courts in the United Kingdom. With a background working with children and families, Jenice has also appeared as Guest Lecturer with the National Youth Services in her native Jamaica. In March 2014, she was welcomed by the Jamaica Association of Social Workers (JASW) and has since been invited to participate in their month-long events in celebration of Social Work Month 2014. Jenice was also interviewed on Jamaica's prominent radio station, *Power 106 FM.*

Jenice recently won the title **"Best Author" in the BEFFTA Awards 2015**, for her second book, ***Damn It, I'm Worthy: 7 Steps to Transform the Relationship with Yourself***, which showcases her energy and passion for owning our self-worth and our individual journeys to healing and self-love. She is also the author of ***Immigrant Workers to the UK: A Personal Journey to Success,*** being featured in The Voice Newspaper (UK) and appearing as a guest contributor to Migration Pulse Publication (UK). As a Jamaican immigrant to the United Kingdom, she shares her experience and engages persistently in dynamic discussions on immigration throughout the UK.

As someone who has successfully moved through

sexual trauma to become a sexually empowered woman, Jenice passionately supports singles and couples in the development of their own sexual confidence and the empowerment of their sexual selves. She works with both men and women to empower their sexual identity and to develop a relationship with the sexual self, giving them the confidence to express, celebrate, and fully enjoy their sexual identity and find pleasurable satisfaction.

WWW.JENICEREVERS.COM
INFO@JENICEREVERS.COM

Lightning Source UK Ltd.
Milton Keynes UK
UKOW04f0920190116

266671UK00002B/21/P

9 780993 515606